From Wu Chi to Tai Chi

A Story of Ancient Beginnings

Richard Leirer

Qigong Academy Press
Ranchos de Taos, New Mexico
2012

Qigong Academy Press
PO BOX 2524
Ranchos de Taos, NM 87557
www.RichardLeirer.org

Copyright ©2012 by Richard Leirer
Second edition ©2013.

13   12   11   10   9

ISBN 978-0-9885478-1-0

1. From Wu Chi to T'ai Chi 1. Title

Table of Contents

Acknowledgements

A special thank you to Jeannie Koran for taking pictures, posing for movements and most importantly, for encouraging me to write. Thank you Mary Cuchna for getting the Tai Chi and Qigong directions organized. Thank you Annya Whalen for editing and structural feedback. Thank you Marie for your editing help. Thank you David for your support and inspiration. Allison, your help with the front cover and graphic design brought the book together.

To my children: Amy, Eric, Lisa and Jonathan, I hope you find inspiration in this book in many ways. Love, Dad.

To my students: You have been a joy in my life, and I treasure each and every class we have had together. I hope this book helps you on your journey.

To my teachers and masters: I hear your words and voices in my inner dialogue. You have helped me become a more loving, caring and gentle person. With deep gratitude and appreciation, I give a bow.

Author's Notes

This is a story of the ancient philosophical beginnings of Qigong and Tai Chi development in China. It is designed as a framework for using Tai Chi /Qigong as tools to develop the consciousness needed for a lifetime of individual self-cultivation. This cultivation leads to increased health, longevity and the possibility of enlightenment. It begins with the ancient concept of Wu Chi and flows forward to cover the emerging world of Tai Chi and all of its tenets.

Through my personal years of research, I discovered that ancient Chinese sages found ways to break through the patterns of conditioned dysfunctional thinking using Qigong and Tai Chi practice. For them Qigong and Tai Chi practice is more than simple health maintenance. It is a profound way to live.

Sage Kuei -Shan Ling -Yu (771 – 853) said:

" If one has true awakening …there are still habitual tendencies that have accumulated over numberless kalpas (life times) which cannot be purified in a single instant. That person should be taught how to gradually remove the karmic tendencies and mental habits. "

(Cheng Chen Bhikshu p. 25)

Families pass on karmic tendencies and mental habits which we pick up and embrace. Changing those conditioned patterns is called cultivation. A cultivation of the mind, body and spirit. The Chinese call these the Jing, the Chi, and the Shen. Jing is the form, Chi is the energy and Shen is the spirit. This book is a **How To Manual** for breaking the conditioned patterns that bind us to a way of being. This is a book about freedom to be what you are naturally. This is about aligning with the cosmic forces and allowing the power of the universe to be with you. I hope you come back to it again and again until the chains of conditioning have been released.

Chapter One

Wu Chi - Wuji

無 極

How Everything Started

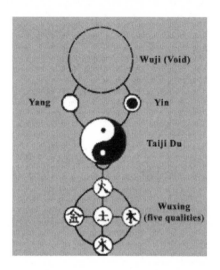

Diagram of the Supreme Ultimate
Created by Chou Tun – Yi (1017 – 1073)

When I began studying Qigong and Tai Chi I was naturally led to Chinese cosmology. I was quickly confused in my study because of language and translation. My teachers in Qigong and Tai Chi would talk about Wu Chi. I did not know what that was and by asking questions. I developed a better understanding. As I began to supplement my training with

1

reading, I became confused by the different spellings I came across in those readings. Is it Wu Chi or Wuji ? And why is it spelled differently? The answer lies in how Chinese language has been translated. Wades-Giles was an early style of translating Chinese words into English and used the spelling Wu Chi. Pinyin is a more modern style of translation, and uses Wuji instead of Wu Chi. You will see this a lot when reading, studying or comparing old translations of Chinese texts or Western books that use one or the other or both of the systems simultaneously. Remember, a rose by any other name will still smell as sweet.

The Rose of Wu Chi is the centerpiece of Chinese cosmology and Qigong Tai Chi practice. Wu Chi is the beginning. In Chinese cosmology it is said that in the beginning, before Heaven and Earth, in the stillness and the void, standing alone and unchanging, was the mother of all things. This was before the Big Bang, before creation, as we know it. The ancient Chinese called this Wu Chi. Wu Chi has always existed and will always exist.

> Wu Chi, a formless state that contains
> all potential existence
> Wu Chi, a formless state that exists before Tai Chi
> Wu Chi, without form, containing the potentiality

of all things even if not yet manifest

The diagram at the beginning of this chapter shows the picture of Chinese Cosmology descending in order of development: from the Wu Chi (the Supreme Ultimate) to the Yin and Yang, which is the Tai Chi, and then to the creation of the five elements that in turn, create all of existence. Wu Chi is a state of existence before anything existed, the ultimate void from which all-else flows. Some Chinese sages say Wu Chi is our home, our original state of existence, before form and body. It is always with us in some metaphysical way, but unless we gain enlightenment, we may never recognize it. Is it the unexplainable place from which we have come and to which we strive to return? Maybe it is what the Christians call heaven. In China, the ancients referred to it as a nothingness that contained everything that has not yet manifest. Wu Chi, to the Qigong and Tai Chi practitioner, is our home and our original and eternal state of existence.

The sages say Tai Chi unfolds from a nothingness that contains everything not yet manifest, waiting for a Yin and Yang expression. This is the way of understanding, say the sages. Does this sound confusing? To Westerners it can; however, to a Chinese mind it may be completely natural. I once had to try and explain the phrase "that's a piece of cake" to my Taiwanese friend Jade. It took a while as she wondered why I used those words to describe an easy task. When I said that it is the easy part of a task, like having cake after a meal she said, "Ohhh, I get it. It's like saying have a piece of fruit." Then I said, "Ohhh, I don't get it." She said, "That's the easy part we eat after the main meal. Our dessert is usually fruit, not cake." This highlighted a cultural difference I had never thought of. As a Westerner, how can I perceive Wu Chi without a cultural awareness of it? Over time and with Qigong practice, I began to develop a greater understanding.

Wu Chi, Yin and Yang, Tai Chi, and the order of the Five Elements are all part of the everyday world for an average Chinese person. These terms are innate to their culture and maybe even their DNA.

It is important for the Western reader unfamiliar with these terms to learn about them to better understand the Qigong/Tai Chi practice. The concept of Chi (Qi) energy, so vital to the practice of Qigong and Tai Chi, is so commonplace in Chinese culture that the daily talk about the weather involves the use of Qi. The very word for weather is Tian Qi or Heaven's Qi. What powerful images come alive when greeting someone and saying something like, "Very nice heaven's Qi we are having today, isn't it?" They speak of a very efficient official or businessperson as having the Qi to get things done (Guan Qi). The Sun is Tai Yang, the big Yang. The language of Qi, Yin and Yang, and Tai Chi is even in the choices and types of food a person eats. Most of us in the West do not have this in-depth cultural exposure to these concepts. A traditional Chinese meal always balances Yin and Yang foods, depending on the seasons and time of the five elements. That is how engrained the concepts are in that society. For Westerners, it is not so matter of fact, and certainly not part of our everyday consciousness. In Adeline Yen Mah's book *Watching the Tree* she tells us that a Chinese language sentence has no need for a verb. This highlights a huge difference in cultural thought.

> In Western thought, subject and attribute are separate. But a sentence such as 'To be or not to be' is impossible to say in Chinese. (I have seen it translated as 'Let me live or let me die'). In the West, existence is thought of as an independent attribute that can be added or subtracted from a separate form. The Chinese language does not separate the two. A simple English sentence such as 'There is a dog' would be translated into Chinese as 'Has dog'… There is no exact Chinese equivalent to 'is'. (Mah p.188-189)

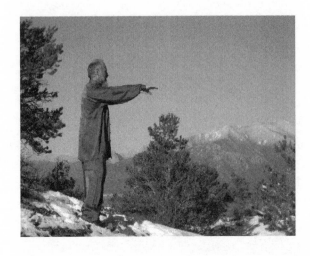

Opening Tai Chi Movement

Again, language and culture are obstacles in developing a clearer understanding of Qigong/Tai Chi principles. The very first movement in all Tai Chi forms sets this Cosmological philosophical experience of moving from Wu Chi to Tai Chi into motion. As competitive as the different Tai Chi styles can be, this is an area all forms agree upon. The opening movement must always represent the transition from the Wu Chi state to the Tai Chi state.

Understanding the depths of these words will bring a clearer understanding of how to perform the Tai Chi forms, and why.

The idea of an existence before existence, i.e. Wu Chi, can appear to be a play of words. What if it is not? Could this be a description of what cannot be adequately described and what might be considered indescribable, and yet able to be experienced?

Knowing how difficult it is to talk of such things, ancient sages used poems and stories to educate. Lao Tzu was such a sage. He wrote the poems of the *Tao Te Ching*.

In Chapter 25 of the *Tao Te Ching* as translated by Gia-Fu Feng and Jane English, Lao- Tzu speaks of not knowing by name, but by actuality.

> Something mysteriously formed,
>
> Born before heaven and earth.
>
> In the silence and the void,
>
> Standing alone and unchanging,
>
> Ever present and in motion.
>
> Perhaps it is the mother of ten thousands things.
>
> I do not know its name.
>
> Call it Tao.

Lao Tzu tries to educate us about an origin and says we can call it a name. He calls it Tao, translated usually as "the way." However, he knows that words are unable to describe what cannot be described, so he writes:

The Tao that can be told is not the eternal Tao.

The name that can be named is not the eternal name.

The nameless is the beginning of heaven and earth.

The named is the mother of ten thousands things.

(Chapter one of the *Tao Te Ching* as translated by Gia-

Fu Feng and Jane English)

Lao Tzu tells us that as we name something, it loses its originality and is locked into a specific idea. In order to discuss something, we need words. Remember, they are just words and words can never accurately describe the indescribable. However, something can be pointed to, therefore words are used to point to the beginning. In the Christian Bible cosmology, Genesis 1 says "In the beginning God created the heavens and the earth. Now the earth was a formless void."

In Chinese cosmology, the beliefs about the creation of the Universe begin with the concept of the nameless Wu Chi or the void. This is a time and place that hold the potential for all things, but has not yet manifested into anything. The Wu Chi is first written about in the *Book of Changes* or *I Ching*. It is said in the "Ta Chuan" or Great Treatise:

In the I Ching (Appendix III) says: In the I there is the Great Ultimate (t'ai Chi 太極), which produced the two forms (i), or Liung Yi. Those two forms generate the four emblems of Ssu Hsiang, and those four emblems produced the eight trigrams or Pa Kua." (Yu-Lan vl p.385).

Wu Chi or Hsien Chi means, "what there is before the universe comes into being." This is also referred to as the Subtle Origin. In the *Hua Hu Ching* :

It was revealed that the developing universe is the expression of its subtle nature, which is the same reality as the subtle truth of being and non-being and the subtle law of all existence and non existence... The development of the universe is its own law, its own reason and its own way as the totality of one life. Therefore, to the narrative mind it is unnamable and beyond description. In other words, by looking at the outer physical universe and its movements one can discover the physical universe and its mechanisms. With developed vision, spiritually developed ones can see the law, the truth, reason and way of the self-born, self-operating, self-generating and regenerating essence of the multi-natural world and use simple language to call it 'Tao.' (Ni p.169)

Tao is used to describe the natural unfolding of existence, including the Wu Chi state. Tao does not exist sometime or somewhere else, but is everywhere and at all times now. Sometimes ancient Chinese authors used the word Tao and Wu Chi interchangeably. That is part of the difficulty in translating from a different culture. (See my chapter 7 on Tao for more detail.)

In an emergence from nothing to something, there is always a now. This now reveals a truth that can be difficult to understand. To understand this truth we need to observe this Tao, understand its principles, and learn from what it offers. Through this observation of now comes an understanding that there is a conditioning that affects all that happens, as well as the recognition that there is a beyond, or before, conditioned consciousness. The conditioned consciousness is known as Tai Chi, and the unconditioned consciousness is known as Wu Chi. Wu Wei is a termed used to describe effortless action, free from conditioning. Wu Wei is a state of " Flow" that brings about effortless action and comes from the connection to the Wu Chi consciousness.

After the Universe came into being from the Wu Chi, a concept of time and existence became present and it was called the Tai Chi. The Tai Chi involved a movement of expansion and contraction of the forces of Yin and Yang. The Wu Chi is always present, yet we normally are not aware of it and cannot contact with it in the normal waking state. Tai Chi is the state of opposites that we are in constant contact with. Tai Chi is the state of existence that we normally live in, usually not in a balanced fashion. This lack of balance is the root of illness and discontent, and pushes us further and further away from effortless action. A more balanced Tai Chi state moves us closer and closer to effortless action and connection with the Wu Chi. That is one reason to practice the Qigong and Tai Chi. These practices create balance and are a road or pathway to Wu Chi.

In a way, Wu Chi is the essence of my pure self. It is the potential of unlimited possibilities of what I can say, or do with my life. Tai Chi becomes what I finally actually do. Within each person is the original pure self, like the original pure subtle origin of Wu Ji. This is the unconditioned self, buried, yet always present in the conditioned self. This original self wants to be freed from the chains of the conditioning that have occurred since birth. The conditioned self wants to follow the conditioned path and to do what we were told to do by parents and teachers. We become who we were told to be, and lose our original nature. Acting in a particular way and being a good boy or girl is constantly drilled into our psyches. We are instructed to follow a particular religion or philosophy as part of a cultural or ethnic identity. We all have been programmed into society, and that program is what we all experience. The self that was created as a response to all that programming becomes the current existence. All dysfunctional behavior lies within this conditioning. Freedom from that programmed thinking lies in finding the unconditioned true self, or the Wu Chi state of existence. Gaining even a small glimpse of this Wu Chi can have a lifelong effect on how we see the universe around us. The ability to experience equanimity of all that is, if even for a second, can be a reward that will last a lifetime.

That is why Master Ni says:

> With developed vision, spiritually developed ones can see the law, the truth, reason and way of the self born, self operating, self generating and regenerating essence of the mind of the multi natural world and use simple language to call it Tao.

The goal in Tai Chi and Qigong cultivation is to find the true self (free from conditioning) and remove the old habits and conditioning that stop the true self from emerging. As children, many of us were scolded with, "Who do you think you are?" or similar messages that stopped the natural development of the self. As children, we quickly learned to adapt or change our natural behavior to please others. In doing so, we lost our original self and have suffered ever since.

Ken Wilber devotes an entire chapter towards "Two Modes of Knowing" in his *The Spectrum of Consciousness*. I believe he is accurately describing the Wu Chi and Tai Chi states of consciousness. He states that our consciousness is split from a primary mode of knowing (Wu Chi) into a dualistic (Tai Chi) mode of knowing. He quotes the biophysicist L.L. Whyte as saying man "has created two worlds from one." (Wilber p.75)

He continues:

> It is precisely in the dualism of 'creating two worlds from one' that the universe becomes severed, mutilated, and consequently 'false to itself,' as G. Spencer Brown pointed out. And the very basis of

this 'creating two worlds from one' is the dualistic illusion that the subject is fundamentally separate and distinct from the object. As we have seen, this is exactly the insight that these physicists had stumbled upon, the culminating insight of three hundred years of persistent and consistent scientific research. Now this is of the utmost importance, for these scientists could realize the inadequacy of dualistic knowledge only by recognizing (however dimly) the possibility of *another mode of knowing* Reality, a mode of knowing that does not operate by separating the knower and the known, the subject and the object.

This is the primary goal of Qigong/Tai Chi: To use one-pointedness of concentration on the form being performed, be it a movement set or a meditation set, through active attention, factors Two and Three emerge. This is the practice of the return to Wu Chi. Most of us live in the Tai Chi realm of conditioning and have lost the ability to have effortless action because that action is overridden by our conditioning.

In ancient China this mode of knowing was called Wu Chi. To take action in this state is known as Wu Wei, or effortless action.

Effortless action does not mean to do nothing. It means to take appropriate action according to the eternal now. Ancient sages have indicated that to live in this state of existence is our goal, our awakening. Modern psychologists suggest the same.

How is this mode of knowing made known? According to Wilber:

> **Factor One**: Active Attention. A special type of intense yet relaxed alertness.
>
> **Factor Two**: Stopping or the suspension of unwanted thought, of conceptualizations, of objectification, of mental chatter. Stopping is in fact, the suspension of the first mode of knowing, of the dualistic and symbolic map knowledge that ultimately distorts reality. In short this is the stopping of the Primary Dualism.
>
> **Factor Three**: Finally there can emerge a Choice less awareness – a special seeing... true seeing and eternal seeing...it operates without any effort whatsoever." (Wilber p.345)

Original being is one unified existence with all things. Original being is not separate in any way from anything. My original being is always a part of the Wu Chi. However by identifying with only myself, I have lost my awareness of my oneness with everything, and I have instead entered into a state of separation of self from everything else. Qigong and Tai Chi are methods of reconnecting with oneness. They are tools to recreate this primordial connection and way of being. That connection happens through concentration.

The diagram at the opening of this chapter also shows the cosmology of Wu Chi to Tai Chi to the *Wu Xing* or Five Elements. The five elements of wood – fire – earth – metal, and water, come into play after the separation into the Tai Chi from the Wu Chi. These elements represent an order in creation. The Yin and Yang of the Tai Chi are two, one Yin and one Yang. Add another Yin or Yang and you have three units of a combination of Yin or a Yang. It is from these three that all form is created. The ancient Chinese sage Chou Tun-Yi states:

> The five elements come into being each having its own particular nature. The true substance of the ultimateless (Wu Chi), and the essence of the two forms (Tai Chi) and the five elements (Wu Xing), unite in mysterious union, so that consolidation ensues. The Yin & Yang by their interaction operate

to produce all things, and these in their turn produce
and reproduce, so that transformation and change
continue without end. (Fung YuLan v2. p.437)

In the *Tao Te Ching*, Lao Tzu describes creation as:

> Tao gives life to the one
> The one gives life to the two
> The two gives life to the three
> The three give life to ten thousand things
> All beings support yin and embrace yang
> And the interplay of these two forces
> Fills the universe.
>
> (Ch 42: Jonathan Star Translation)

Study of the *I Ching* and Chinese Traditional Medicine is needed for further explanation of the complexities of the five elements and Yin and Yang. My chapter 3 on Tai Chi is a primer in understanding some parts of this complexity. Note that in advanced internal Qigong practice we need to work with two of these five primal elements, fire and water, to recreate our original nature. This involves an advanced form of concentration called the merger of Kan and Li. Before attempting that higher level of cultivation practice, we have to first work with the Yin and Yang through our Qigong Tai Chi practice. (See my chapter 4 on Te for further information on the Kan and Li.)

The important thing to remember about Wu Chi in Chinese Cosmology is that it is like talking about heaven to a Christian.

Wu Chi is the experience the Chinese sage hopes to have, and heaven is the goal for the Christian. In Qigong and Tai Chi, the goal is enlightenment and is the ultimate purpose behind all of the practice and is manifest as as a return to the Wu Chi state of existence. Wu Chi is the state of my original existence.

In China, I studied a special Wu Chi Qigong set with the late master Zhu Wei from Tien Tai Mountain. Modern Qigong practitioners sometimes translate Wu Chi as "primordial." While performing these movements, I wondered how this movement would ever bring me to a primordial state of awareness. Only by recognizing that Wu Chi always exists did I come to understand why the practice was created. We need to be reminded of our origins, and a physical reminder is needed to help the consciousness of our cells remember what existed before form. Sometimes "just doing" a movement creates a level of awareness words cannot express. It is like looking at nature or a piece of art or hearing beautiful music. Just experiencing these things creates a change of consciousness.

The concept of consciousness in ancient Chinese culture is bound with the Shen (Xin), or spirit. The Westerner usually sees consciousness as a structure of the mind, a part of the physical body. My masters recognized that we have a chemical encoding in our body that can be called consciousness. However our real consciousness is beyond body and lives in our shen or spirit. Our shen is embodied in our Qi. The Qi is embodied in our physical form. The area of the physical heart is where the shen consciousness is primarily centered. Sometimes this consciousness is translated as Heart-Mind. Often times the heart is highly emotionally charged. This emotional charge prevents our wisdom mind form being activated. Master Yang Jwing-Ming says our emotional mind is like an ape and our wisdom mind is like a horse. We can tame a monkey mind with a banana. The equivalent of a banana for our emotional mind is the breath. Breath work helps us to tame our monkey mind and allows our wisdom mind to develop. Strong and stable, like a horse.

> This banana is in control of the breathing. As long
> as you are able to concentrate your mind on your
> breathing, sooner or later your emotional mind will

be restrained and calm down. (Jwing-Ming p. 80)

The advanced art of cultivation is to use the body to recognize the Qi, to use the Qi to recognize the shen or spirit, and to use the spirit to recognize the Wu Chi origin. This is what the ancients referred to as changing Jing into Qi (*Lian Jing Hua Qi* (精化气)), changing Qi into spirit (*Lian Qi Hua Shen* (炼气化神)), returning spirit to nothingness (*Lian Shen Huan Xu* (炼神还虚)), and combining nothingness with Tao, (*Lian Xu He Dao* (炼虚合道)). Through this reversal of awareness, a person becomes *Shen Ren* (精神的人), or a spirit person who has returned to Wu Chi.

In the late 1600's Chinese scholars Huang Tsung-Yen and Chu Yi-Tsun stated the Diagram of the Supreme Ultimate was originally called "The Diagram of the Ultimateless" (*Wu Chi Tu*), and that a diagram by that name is carved on the face of a cliff in Hua Shan. At the bottom of the diagram is a circle labeled "Doorway of the Mysterious Female." (See *Tao Te Ching* Ch. 06 for other references to the mysterious female) The mysterious female is the "Base From Which Heaven and Earth Sprang," Above this circle on the carving is still another circle with the inscriptions of "*Lian Jing Hua Qi, Lian Qi Hua Shen* and *Lian Xu He Dao*." (Fung Yu Lan v2. 441)

This is the ancient formula for returning to the Tao or Wu Chi and the state of enlightenment. Finding a teacher is needed in order to follow this formula to completion. Using a book or video will not work.

The spiritual practice of a Chinese sage is one of spiritual or internal alchemy. Neigong Qigong, is the internal practices of this alchemy.

The first step in this alchemical transformation is the recognition of the Qi energy that permeates all form, including the human body.

This is the meaning of the words *Lian Jing Hua Qi*. This is the first stage in cultivation. The goal is to transform jing or original energy into form or matter energy. It is the recognition of the Qi energy that permeates the body.

The second stage is direct awareness of the spirit (shen) consciousness that is the ever present "I " that lives inside the physical form. This "I "awareness is always present. However he essence of this "I" becomes more direct from intense awareness of the Qi in the body and the mental connection with the Qi energy.

Awareness of Qi energy in our meditations or during our Tai Chi and

Qigong practice reveals the existence of the spirit or the consciousness of the always present "I "observer. This is the second stage of cultivation called *Lian Qi Hua Shen*. This experience of the shen frees us from the attachment to the body. It is an experience that lets us know we are more then body and helps to release the attachment to form.

The last stage in our cultivation is to return our spirit to the Tao of everythingness. This is the complete return to Wu Chi.

Wuji means 'No Extremity,' and means
'No Dividing' or 'No Discrimination.'

Wuji is a state of formlessness, of staying in the center:
calm, quiet, and peaceful.

Once you have generated a mind, or have formed the
mental shape with which you will influence physical
reality, the motivation of dividing or discriminating starts.
When this dividing happens, Wuji will be derived into
Yin and Yang. From this, you learn what Taiji is – it is the
motivation of distinguishment.

When you have this motivation, the Qi will then be led,
and Yin and Yang can be distinguished.

Dr. Yang, Jwing-Ming   June 06, 2011

Richard Leirer

Chapter 2

Li

理

The Function or Principle
That Underlies Everything

Finding purpose in life is a major theme for many. What will I do? What type of career will I have? How will I spend my day? What will I do in my day? How do I find out what I am good at? What is the meaning of my life anyway? These are all questions asked by many at one time or another in a life. Chinese philosophy says the ultimate goal is to return to the original source of Wu Chi. For that to happen it will be helpful to discover the Li of your life. Li is the function or principle that underlies everything, including your life. The famous Chinese Historian Fung Yu Lan tells us:

> The Supreme Ultimate lacks shape but contains Principle (Li). Because this principle is multiple, therefore physical objects are also multiple. Without a particular principle or Li, no given object can

25

exist...For all things created in the universe there
is in each a particular principle. (Fung v.1 p.535)

There is a principle that underlies everyone's life and everything in life. Discovering what that principle is can take a lifetime. For some, it changes as parts of their life change. As a child our function is different from that of an adult. An employer's function is different from that of an employee.

Understanding the Li of Qigong and Tai Chi is essential for enlightenment and awakening. Understanding the function, or Li, of Qigong/Tai Chi health benefits is helpful, as is knowing the martial arts applications or principles of a movement.

This principle, or Li, comes from the Wu Chi, and it is what is inherently *natural* for all that exists. The Wu Chi contains the essence of all things, including its principle function and the not yet manifest. The Wu Chi is the void of unlimited potentials, and the Tai Chi is the present dualistic realm of existence. Tai Chi is what exists now and is perceived in a dualistic or dialectic fashion. Wu Chi and Tai Chi interact with each other, and they do so in an orderly way through the natural function of Li. The Wu Chi is never really gone, only unacknowledged. It is like having a present thought. Did that thought exist before it was thought? The answer is yes. The potential for the thought is always within the thinker. It simply was not yet made manifest. For whatever reason, the thought does come into being, and now it is present as an emergence from nothing into something. The Tai Chi, also, is an emergence of something from nothing. The movement from Wu Chi, or void, into something is the act of Tai Chi. My potential is my Wu Chi; my actions are my Tai Chi. Li is the inherent function of all. What is the function of Qigong/Tai Chi? The answer is many functions, with the ultimate one being enlightenment or awakening to our true and original nature and purpose in life.

The idea of constant change rules the concept of Tai Chi. The Li or principle of all things contains a Yin and Yang of potential change. This combining of apparent opposites, which form a whole, is known as Tai Chi, or the embrace of Yin and Yang. Yin is action that is inward, downward, and condensing. Yang is action that is outward, opening, and expanding. This combination of Yin and Yang always forms something new and is an act of creation. This something new is similar to the Hegelian Dialectic of Thesis-Antithesis-Synthesis. This is the fundamental principle for Yin and Yang.

The Li of the hair on a horse is to protect and serve the horse when it is on the horse. That same hair, when removed from the horse and made into a paintbrush, now has a different Li, the Li of a paintbrush. I can change my Li from how I was raised into the Li of what I want to become. If I change and allow my natural self to be present, my natural Li will also become manifest. I can become awakened to a new creation, a new person, and my natural self. That new person is what the Chinese call *Shen Ren*, or spirit person and is the ultimate goal of the Qigong/Tai Chi practitioner. Physical, mental, emotional and spiritual skills are developed with practice that brings about this transformation.

Li comes from what we do and who we believe we are. Our beliefs change over time and with influence from others and our practice. Yet each of us has an original Li or an original nature that is an extension of the Wu Chi. Like the original hair on a horse's back, that hair can change from a horse's coat to become a paintbrush. I, as a person, can also change over time and become who I was naturally born to be.

Change always takes place in some way, and our Li changes with us. However, our original self contains the unchanging purpose of our existence, the how and why of our being. Tai Chi reminds us that as we develop into our original selves, who we are changes, and what we are always remains the same. We are a part of the Wu Chi and have never really been separated from it. The apparent separation is the basis of Tai Chi. When something comes into existence, that is the Tai Chi set in motion.

In all Qigong and Tai Chi practice there is a Li, or function, operating within the practice. Understanding how the body moves in a particular way is a function. Knowing how the energy flows in a movement is a function. Knowing the application of a movement is a function. Think about the function of a knife. It is to cut. What is the function of a gun? What is the function of your practice? What is the function of your awareness or attention? This is important in training. In Qigong/Tai Chi it is important to know the function of the practice. In Tai Chi forms, it is important to know both the application and the energy patterns and flow. It is important to know which part of the movement is Yin and which is Yang. Where do they meet? How do they merge? One must know the Li of the practice.

When I was a teenager and just beginning my cultivation, I studied Martial Arts with the American Kung Fu and Karate Federation. My Sifu, master Guy Savelli, taught us many martial applications and methods of mental awareness. He had a saying: "Never put yourself in a position to be beat." This meant always be aware of your surroundings and pay attention to potential danger. What it created within me and other students was a background paranoia in which I was constantly aware of potential dangers. The Li, or function, was to be hyper-vigilant at all times.

This training took place in Cleveland, Ohio during the Viet Nam war era. It would have been very helpful if I were at war in Viet Nam, and it also was somewhat helpful growing up in the inner city, a place of potential danger. It created within me a young man who was ready and able to defend himself. That was the function of the training. Unfortunately, even when there was no danger, I still wanted to express my skills at martial arts. I began to look for potential danger or even create it myself with lines like "who you looking at?" or "you want a piece of this?" My function, or Li, was the product of my training, which was out of balance. Within a short while (three years), I was able to see the dangers of this Li and adjust my training towards healing. That meant finding a new teacher who provided training in a different way.

George Clooney made a movie called *The Men Who Stare at Goats.* Although the movie was created to be a comedy, it was about a real experiment that the US military did with Sifu Savelli and others. The movie title comes from Savelli's ability to stare, or project his Qi, into a goat, until the goat became unconscious. Savelli was at one end of the barracks and the goat at the other end and he was able to influence the heart rate of the goat, dropping the goat's heart rate until it became unconscious. This experiment was part of a movement by the U.S. military to create new warriors and access the mysteries of Qi for military gain.

While I am grateful for the training I received from Sifu Savelli, I also realized the dangers of this type of practice, and the person I was becoming as a result of practicing with him. The Li was for death and killing and destruction. Although I stopped my training with him before the goat experiment was conducted, I learned his techniques for accomplishing this task. Later I was able to harness the same Qi for healing work. This represents the duality of training. The mental concentration and Qi projection needed to accomplish this task can easily be translated to healing energy instead of deadly energy.

My hope is that others who practice Qigong and Tai Chi become aware of the Li behind their practice and notice what that Li is creating within. When the practice is used for health, longevity and enlightenment, you can never go wrong. Remember:

The principle or Li of a thing is the all perfect form

or supreme archetype of that thing. (Fung v.1 537)

We need to find that all perfect form within ourselves. Tai Chi is translated as Supreme Ultimate. That translation comes about because the word Tai has a base meaning of great or supreme and Chi has the meaning of containing the "ultimate" Li. The next chapter reveals the hidden meaning of Tai Chi as a means for awakening that natural Li within.

Chapter 3

Tai Chi or TaiJi
Yin and Yang

太極

The Always Changing Environment

When I began my martial arts training I really did not care what the Li of the practice was. I wanted to learn how to do what David Carradine did in the *Kung Fu* TV series. What an awesome TV program that led many like me to seek the ancient Chinese Way of life! After many years of practice I did learn that the principle, or Li, of Tai Chi is to create a balance of Yin and Yang energies. Tai Chi is also used to describe the interaction of energy patterns that remain constant in all of existence. Through observation, the ancients noticed a dialectic exchange taking place within all form, including within each individual. The Li of the Yin and the Yang in everything became evident.

Within form, or the Tai Chi Realm, there is a part appearing to stay the same and a part apparently changing. There is a part that is still, and a part that is active. There is a part that is Yin, which is close or near, and a part that is Yang, which is far or distant. Tai Chi is the up side and the down side, and the inside and the outside of everything that exists.

In simple terms, Tai Chi has also been described as the sunny side of the hill and the shadow side. In more complex terms, it is said that "Tai Chi is what lies within shapes and features." The Wu Chi is "what lies beyond shapes and features." (Fung v.1 p.94)

Wu Chi is a state of existence from which potential thought arises. Tai Chi is the present thought I have within myself. If I find I have a thought, I may ask where it came from. Usually, what I think is my own thought is actually a thought from someone else. Look at children and see how they mimic their parents in both words and deeds. Those words and deeds do not really change so much from parent to child.

Our response to a stimulus usually has a root in our conditioning. The way and manner in which I was raised is instilled within me, and I act accordingly. As a result of my early training, I am unable to respond naturally to the world around me because my conditioned Li has replaced my original natural Li. I have encoded the so-called proper responses from my parents, brothers and sisters, and teachers. Thus,

I have enslaved myself to the thoughts of others. I have become out of balance and away from my natural self, or balanced Tai Chi self.

When I speak from my own heart, with my own thoughts, and engage in the world around me without the constant demand to follow the ideas of others, I am more in a state of original balanced Tai Chi. This balance has been measured by modern research and demonstrates that those who practice Qigong and Tai Chi actually use their brain waves in a more balanced fashion than non Tai Chi practitioners.

The research of Dr. Shin Lin, P.H.D shows that:

> Pilot experiments involving electroencephalography (EEG) were conducted in collaboration with Dr. Ramesh Srinivasan at the Cognitive Science Department of University of California, Irvine, and with Dr. Tzyy-Ping Jung at the Swartz Center for Computational Neuroscience of the University of California, San Diego (12). A number of experienced Qigong and Tai Chi practitioners were recorded with a 128-channel EEG system (Geodesic Sensor Net System from Electrical Geodesic, Inc.) before, during,

and after meditation in the sitting position. With highly experienced subjects, there was an increase in alpha and theta waves recorded at the frontal mid-line area of the head within minutes into the meditative period compared to the baseline level recorded before and after this period. When the EEG data were further examined by the method of Independent Component Analysis (14), we found that the increase in alpha and theta waves was also accompanied by an increase in beta waves (12,13). Since alpha and theta waves signify a state of relaxation and rest while beta waves reflect a state of alert consciousness, this analysis indicates that meditation is a dual state of 'relaxed concentration.' (For Dr. Sin Lin's complete report see Appedix p. 219)

This conclusion indicates Qigong and Tai Chi practitioners have an effective way to train the mind to be sharply focused during mental activities in every day life. Through the practice of Qigong/Tai Chi, the function of the brain changes into a "relaxed concentration" state, thereby allowing the natural Li to emerge. As a result of my practice I have become a happier, healthier and more loving person. I have discovered the strength of softness that comes from Qigong/Tai Chi practice.

Tai Chi and Yin and Yang Theory

It was said that watching the workings of sun and shadow on the two opposite sides of a pagoda or the sides of a hill brought a clear understanding of Yin and Yang. When the sun was shining on one side, the other was dark with shadow. After a while, the shadow side became the sun side, and the sun side fell into shadow. The observation of this interplay of light and dark gave rise to the understanding of the nature of constant change from Yin to Yang and Yang back to Yin. It also allowed for the realization that all things are relative to the observer and the manner in which information is perceived.

Chinese Traditional Medical Theory holds the premise that the body, particularly the organs and acupuncture channels, is in a constant state of paired workings of Yin and Yang. This allows the human body to maintain health and balance. Excess of Yin and/or Yang in one or more organs or acupuncture channels has to be compensated for by other parts of the body, or health cannot be maintained.

Yin and Yang theory is represented by the *Tai Chi Tu*, or diagram, that shows a circle with what appears to be two fish connected to each other, one dark and the other white. This symbol is widely recognized throughout the world today, but few recognize the complexity of its meaning.

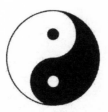

Within the concept of Yin and Yang exists a basic premise: There is in the Universe an energy source that gathers and manifests itself in subjective reality through the concept of Yin and Yang. This basic energy structure is called Qi (Chi). Without Qi, there is no life.

Remember that in Chinese Cosmology, in the beginning was the state of emptiness, or void (Wu Chi). This is the Tao producing the one as mentioned in the Tao Te Ching, quoted on page 18.

The one (Wu Chi) gives life to the two or Tai Chi and the Yin and Yang of everything. The two (Tai Chi) continue to merge until all elements are created giving life to the three energies of all elements. The three (all elements) continue to merge until the form of all of existence is established (the ten thousand things).

Tai Chi is both a Qigong practice and an idea about the constantly changing modes of observing perceptions of reality. The Tai Chi contains an active integration. Yin represents the less changing, still, near, solid, female aspects of observation. Yang represents greater changing, moving, far, gaseous, and male aspects. Tai Chi forms are choreographed to create a balance in the body by the nature of the movement. When a movement is performed, it takes mental concentration and the physical firing of electrical charges from nerves to muscles to perform the action. Ideally, that action will create a balance between the physical body and the mental component of the movement, and harmonize the acupuncture channels in the body, which are stimulated as a result of the movement. This is why Tai Chi is so beneficial to the human body, thereby creating great health.

The great teacher Lao has said, "A single Yin cannot be born, and a single Yang cannot be grown." This means that Yin and Yang are not tangible things. They are just observable ways to describe something, regardless of what that something is. The practice of Tai Chi and Qigong, then, is a practice of an idea and a method of balance.

In the same way that mathematics is an expression or language of symbols, Tai Chi expresses the language of the dialectic. It is a concept that is used as an observation method of two phenomena. An essential point is that the position of the observer influences the relationship of Yin and Yang in the comparison of objects. To illustrate this principle, we can describe the Earth as Yin and the moon as Yang. From the point of view of an observer on Earth, the Earth is near and the moon is far. However, if we compare the moon to the sun using the same criteria of near/far, the moon becomes Yin and the sun becomes Yang. Now compare the sun to the galaxy. Which is Yin or Yang? See how the sun becomes Yin in that comparison.

Compare our galaxy to the universe: which is Yin and which is Yang? Tai Chi is relative because Yin and Yang are relative. There is always some Yin within Yang. That is why the Tai Chi symbol has both a white dot within the black fish and vice versa. Yin can be said to be still when compared to movement, which is Yang. Yang can be said to be up as compared to Yin, which is down. The Moon can be said to be Yang when compared to the Earth. However when compared to the Sun, it becomes Yin. Upward movement can be said to be Yang movement, and downward can be said to be Yin movement. My upbringing and my experiences can be called Yin. My actions and words can be called Yang. In Tai Chi practice, the outward moving part of a movement is Yang, and the inflowing part is Yin.

Within each individual Yin and Yang are in constant change. At a basic level, it can be said that a person is part earth (Yin) and part heaven (spirit or Yang). What is from earth will return to earth; what is from heaven (spirit or Shen) will return to heaven. Humankind is, thus, the embodiment of Tai Chi, being part earth and part heaven.

There are also levels of Tai Chi within the body: interior/exterior, Yin organs/Yang organs, Yin acupuncture channels/Yang acupuncture channels, and so forth. It is even noted that our spirit is Yin/Yang. The ancient Chinese sages have named the two differing parts of our spirit the Hun and the Po. The earthly part of our spirit, or Hun, wants to continue with all the earthly experiences. Meanwhile, the heavenly part of our spirit, or Po, wants to return to its original home, the Wu Chi, or the Return to the One. Chinese Taoists believe that there are seven realms of consciousness in the Tai Chi Realm and two states of consciousness in the Wu Chi Realm. Only after transcending all nine realms can we truly go home to the Wu Chi.

Tai Chi can also be expressed as a function of our consciousness or our ability to think. In the West, this is often called the conscious and the unconscious. In Chinese philosophy, this concept is known as the conditioned mind and the unconditioned mind. The conditioned mind is said to occur after leaving heaven or Wu Chi and entering into the Tai Chi realm of existence. The Tai Chi realm is the collection of information accumulated through the senses, and is also called the carved block. Jung called this carved block the collective unconscious. The state known as the uncarved block is the state of a person's consciousness before birth.

Jung says:

> Observations made in my practice have opened me to quite new and unexpected approach to Eastern wisdom... I have been unconsciously led along that secret way which has been the preoccupation of the best minds of the East for centuries...The psyche possesses a common substratum transcending all differences in culture and consciousness. I have called this substratum the collective unconscious. This unconscious psyche, common to all mankind, does not consist merely of contents capable of becoming conscious, but of latent dispositions towards certain identical reactions.
> (Wilhelm, Richard p. 86-87)

Tasting, touching, hearing, seeing and smelling: these impulses have been encoded by our consciousness from a subjective point of view from the moment of conception. This is the beginning of the carving of our block. The meaning assigned to experiences comes from the perception of the viewer. The things we think about have been encoded in conditioned "likes or dislikes." This conditioning leads us to believe that what we experience is good or bad, based on the reinforcement of the belief system. This reinforcement of good and bad comes from our parents, teachers, and society, and can be perceived in any way imaginable. It becomes apparent, however, that family and society influences have the greatest impact on how information is interpreted. In many families, this is how the patterns of dysfunctional behavior are passed on. Conversely, functional behavior can also be passed on.

Through Qigong/Tai Chi practice, the conditioned mind can be deleted or placed into the background, and the unconditioned mind can be activated and brought to the foreground. Sometimes in meditation this is called "sitting and forgetting." Unfortunately, if you try to sit and forget, just the opposite happens. When I did research with veterans suffering from Post-Traumatic Stress Disorder (PTSD), we discovered that clients who just tried to relax and meditate had more time to think of the stressors that created the PTSD. Their minds kept looking back at what happened in their lives, creating more stress, and were unable to clear out the mental chatter and worries. The group that practiced Qigong/Tai Chi did not have this difficulty because their minds had to concentrate on what was being asked of them in order to do the movement. They performed an action that took the mind away from the original stressors and placed their mental attention at the physical level. In this case they were "standing, moving and forgetting." The physical body was relaxing, and the stress-relieving chemicals like serotonin and dopamine were increasing as the result of the practice. The Qigong/Tai Chi practice brought the body back into balance. The stress relief came from working both the unconscious and the conscious mind.

Tai Chi has long been called " meditation in motion." However Harvard Medical School's *Harvard Health Publication* May 2009 issue calls Tai Chi "medication in motion." The article stated that Tai Chi, when combined with standard treatment, is helpful for a range of conditions including arthritis, low bone density, breast cancer, heart disease, heart failure, hypertension, Parkinson's disease, sleep problems, and stroke. That is quite an endorsement of the Li principle of health connected to Tai Chi practice.

Health constitutes a balance of the Yin and Yang in mind as well as body. While under stress we rarely look at the limitless possibilities that might exist. We see only our stressor. Our fixation on our conditioning is the source of most of our stress. What we concentrate on, we see. The balance created by Tai Chi opens the door of awareness to possibilities beyond our conditioning, thereby freeing us from conditioned limitations.

Here is an example from research covered by the New York Times indicating how what we might see is conditioned by societal influence.

Modern Psychology has demonstrated that what a person sees can be predicated on what other people say or do. Famous studies conducted by Dr. Solomon Asch in the 1950's in the United States showed the effect of social conformity in three out of four subjects. In his early experiments subjects were shown two cards. The first had a vertical line and the second had three lines, one of them the same length as that of the first card. The subject were asked to say which two lines were alike, something most 5 yr olds could answer correctly. Unknowing to the subjects, other people in cahoots with Dr.

Asch gave their wrong answers before the subjects gave theirs. Three out of four subjects after hearing this wrong answer also then gave the incorrect answer at least once and one out of four conformed to a wrong answer 50 percent of the time. (Blakeslee, Sandra P. 3, Column 1)

When I was a freshman in High School in 1969 my math instructor performed a similar experiment in which I was a subject. He removed me from the classroom along with two other classmates to the hallway. While we were out in the hallway, he then told the remaining classmates to give an obviously wrong answer when asked to do a math review problem when we came back into the room. He then brought us back in the classroom one by one and asked us to give our math answers after the class gave the wrong answer. My two other classmates, following the lead of the whole class, gave the wrong answer to the math problem after the class said their answer, even though it was obviously not correct.

For me this was very upsetting. I knew what the correct answer was, and I stood by that answer in spite of what my classmates said. I was embarrassed and angry at the teacher and my classmates. The power of the group and the urge to conform was tremendous. I stuck to my guns and did my best to grin and bear it until the teacher told me it was an experiment. The class had a good laugh; I did not. It was very difficult not conforming and going along with the class. This experience became a lesson for me I always remembered. To this day, I am able to see events much more clearly than my friends and family can. The pressure to conform to social norms is great, but not insurmountable. The practice of Qigong/Tai Chi helped me stay more opened and aware of social conditioning.

More modern research echoed the experiment by Dr. Solomon Asch. Dr. Gregory Berns, a neuroscientist at Emory University, says, "Seeing is believing what the group tells you to believe."

In the research published in *Biological Psychiatry* June 22, 2005 subjects participated in similar experiments. This time they had their heads examined, literally, with brain scanners. As before, subjects went along with the wrong answers '41 percent of the time.' The researchers found that there was no activity in brain areas that make conscious decisions for the folks who answered wrongly. As for the other folks who went against the social pressure to conform and actually gave the right answer, they had different parts of their brain activated. The areas associated Dr. Berns says with 'emotional salience.'

(Blakeslee, Sandra p.3)

Even more disturbing is the research titled "Gorillas in our midst: sustained inattentional blindness for dynamic events." The researchers found:

> ...we are surprisingly unaware of the details of our environment from one view to the next: we often do not detect large changes to objects and scenes ('change blindness'). Furthermore, without attention, we may not even perceive objects ('inattentional blindness'). Taken together, these findings suggest that we perceive and remember only those objects and details that receive focused attention. (Daniel J Simons, Christopher F Chabris Department of Psychology, Harvard University, 33 Kirkland Street, Cambridge, MA 02138, USA; Received 9 May 1999, in revised form 20 June 1999.)

In this experiment, subjects did not see a person dressed in a gorilla outfit who walked across an area where others were passing a basketball. The subjects were told to count the number of times the basketball was passed between teammates. With the attention on counting the passing ball, most people literally did not see the gorilla. They were inattentionally blinded by what they were doing. Missing something as absurd and as noticeable as a full size person in a gorilla suit demonstrates the magnitude of events most of us are missing. A video of this experiment and other experiments are available online and you can test yourself. Just Google " Inattentional Blindness" for more up to date research.

Another frightening example of inattentional blindness occurred in similar experiments where airplane pilots in a flight simulator did not see another airplane sitting on a runway while they were landing a plane in simulation. Because it would not normally happen, pilots were blinded to the possibility when it occurred in the experiment. More then 50 percent of the pilots crashed into the parked plane, simply not seeing what was there because the real life experience of a plane being parked on the runway would not normally happen.

The ancients recognized the problem of conditioned response thousands of years ago. In Qigong/Tai Chi practice, the goal is to reach a state of awareness free from conditioning. In the practice of Qigong/Tai Chi, the participant uses concentration on movements and or breathing to let go of the conditioned mind in order to create access to the unconditioned self and to increase awareness. Some of my teachers have referred to this process as Going to the Mountain. Deep relaxed mental concentration creates a slower brain pattern that prepares our consciousness for this experience. Also, concentration training prepares us to engage in "Critical Thinking." This type of thinking bypasses our automatic responses to external stimuli to some degree, and we actually engage in thought, instead of reacting with emotions.

In the original, older Yang and Wu style Tai Chi forms, there is a movement called "Embrace the Tiger, Return to Mountain, Cross Arms." It comes at the end of the first and second circles of the 108 Wu Style Tai Chi. This movement is the physical reminder to embrace our power and return to the mountain before we cross our hands in repose. Our Tiger energy is always present to protect us if need be. Our peaceful, gentle energy is also always present, similar to the feeling a person has when they are in the mountains. If we truly can go to the Mountain in our movement, we have attained great Tai Chi. This Tai Chi knows the fierceness of a Tiger and the gentleness of being in a mountain setting, calm and relaxed. This is the discovery of true power, a power that is both Yin and Yang. Becoming this person is helped by understanding the true meaning of Tai Chi. This true meaning reveals the natural power of

Tai Chi when properly balanced.

If only practiced as a martial art, Tai Chi is not as powerful and this hidden meaning becomes lost.

The Ideogram for Tai Chi and the
True Hidden Meaning of the Characters.

The Characters for Tai Chi are as follows:

Tai 太 and

Chi 極

Tai is usually referred to as great or supreme. Chi (Ji) can be referred to as ultimate. In an article written on Tai Chi Joseph A. Adler explains why Tai Chi means principle (Li):

For example, one of Zhu's prominent disciples was Chen Chun 陳淳 (1159-1223), who wrote (in Wing-tsit Chan's translation): The Great Ultimate simply means principle. Why is principle called ji [極]? Ji means reaching the ultimate, because it is in the center serving as the axis [shuji 樞極]. Huangji [皇極] (royal ultimate), beiji [北極] (the North Pole), etc., all have the meaning of being in the center. But ji should not be understood [literally] as the center. The greatest extent of anything is always in its center. Things from all directions reach their ultimate point here and cannot go any further. Take the ridgepole of a roof. It is called the wuji [屋極]87 (terminus of a building). It is simply the converging point of all building materials from the various directions, reaching their terminus at this center. *On Translating Taiji* by Joseph A. Adler Kenyon College June 2009; revised June 2012

This indicates how the ideogram Tai Chi (Tai Ji) has come to mean Supreme Ultimate or Great Ultimate.

However, another reason it is called Supreme Ultimate is also hidden inside each character and those characters reveal hidden practices. The hidden meaning reveals Tai Chi as more than the idea of a ridge pole or a center place. It refers to the idea of a person becoming One Centered Person, Between Heaven and Earth, Relaxed, Standing like a Pine Tree, Using the Mouth and the Hands in a Balanced Fashion. Here is how to properly read the Chinese Character for its hidden meaning. Look closely at the composite make up of each character.

The first character, 太 Tai, is a combined character composed of three individual characters. First is a straight line meaning one. _____

The second character is a symbol for a person, ren.

人

    ren

—

    The third character is one dot, which represents one or centered.

The hidden meaning of the compound character Tai is One Centered Person Between Heaven and Earth. The head is in heaven and the body is on earth. The mark in the middle indicates the middle or center of the

person, the dan tien. 太 The greatest human achievement is to become a centered and balanced person between heaven and earth. (This is why this character means Supreme.)

The second character is Ji, or Chi. Early Western translations thought this character was the Chi or Qi energy that permeates the universe. The erroneous use of this word came about because the ultimate ideal in Chinese philosophy is the balance of the yin and yang energies that emerge from the Wu Chi. Also because Chi or Qi energy is pronounced similarly and is a key component in Tai Chi practice.

This Ji, or Chi character is another combination word composed of two characters:

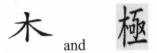 and 極

The character on the left is the character for a tree, in this instance, a pine tree.

木   This tree character refers to the ability to be as relaxed as a pine tree. The word Fang Soong means to be relaxed as a pine tree and is chanted in meditations like *Fang Soong Gong Qigong*. It also refers to the Qigong Tai Chi practice To Stand Like a Tree, sometimes also called Standing Like a Stake or Jam Jhong. This practice allows the Tai Chi practicioner to root into the Yin earth energy and the Yang sky energy, always in a relaxed fashion the way a tree actually does in nature.

The compound character on the right of the character for Ji, or Chi, shows the characters for the hand and mouth contained within two lines and split by a centered line.

口 The mouth character

and the hand character are balanced on each side of each other here on earth.

Notice how the mouth and hand characters are contained between a top line and a bottom line. This indicates on earth, not in heaven. This is the ultimate goal of a person. Having a balanced use of the hand and mouth, here on Earth, using the natural Li or principles inherent within. This is why Ji can be expressed as a "Standard" or an extreme pole to achieve. Adler explains:

> In an exchange on section E of the *Taijitu shuo* and the key term *weifa* (unexpressed [mind]) from the *Zhongyong* 中庸 (The Mean in Practice): Li asked: Are "the reality of the Non-polar" (*wuji zhi zhen* 無極之真) and "the equilibrium of the unexpressed" (*weifa zhi zhong* 未發之中) [mind] the same or different?

> Reply: The reality of the Non-polar includes activity and stillness; the equilibrium of the unexpressed refers only to stillness. *Taiji* is simply the extreme utmost (*jizhi*), but it has no location. [It is] the highest (*zhigao*), the most mysterious (*zhimiao*), the

most essential (*zhijing*), the most spiritual (*zhishen*), [but] with no location. Lianxi [Zhou Dunyi] feared that people would say that *taiji* had form, so he said "*wuji er taiji.*" Within this *wu* there is the principle of the utmost extreme (*zhiji zhi li* 至極之理). It is like *huangji* 皇極 ("royal perfection"), which is the hub of the universe but has no location. It is neither here nor there; it is only at the center, where everything comes together. He then pointed to the peak of the house *wuji* 屋極) and said: It's not even there. (*Yulei* 94:3120).

It is tempting to suspect that in the last sentence Zhu Xi was actually speaking tongue-in-cheek, by pointing to the very object (the ridgepole) that gave *taiji* its root meaning.

'*Huangji*' is a term from the *Hongfan* 洪範 (Great Plan) chapter of the *Shujing* 書經 (Scripture of Documents), where it refers to the ruler as the ultimate standard. In his essay "Analysis of *huangji*" (*Huangji bian*), Zhu says: *Huang* is a designation of the ruler; *ji* means the utmost extreme (*zhi ji* 至極), a name for the norm

57

or standard (*biaozhun* 標準). This is always at the center of a thing, and is what those all around hope to use to rectify themselves. Therefore to take the extreme (*ji*) as the standard (*zhun*) of the center is acceptable, but to take it simply as the center is unacceptable. It is like the North Star as the peak of heaven (*tianji*), or the ridgepole as the peak of a house (*wuji*); their meanings are the same (*Wenji* 72, 3454).

Note that Zhu here does define *ji* as "utmost extreme," which is its colloquial meaning. But as in the previous quote, he combines this with the sense of *ji* as a center – not in a spatial sense, but in a normative sense. This is the aspect of *taiji* that is lost by translating it as "Supreme Ultimate." (Adler p.21)

The characters Tai Chi, or Taiji, literally mean "One Centered Person Between Heaven and Earth Who Knows How to Stand Like a Tree, Be Relaxed as a Pine Tree and Uses the Hand and the Mouth in a Balanced Fashion on Earth." This image is part of Tai Chi cultivation. It is the ideal to strive for. It is the standard to reach.

The Chinese word *Chuan* or *Quan* usually is used in the word for fist or boxing. It is also used in the word earnest or sincere 拳拳 (*Quan Quan*) or " to clasp hands / to put one's palms together (in obeisance) " 擎拳合掌 (*qíngquánhézhǎng*) or "to push up one's sleeves and bare one's fists / to be eager to get started " 捋臂揎拳 (*luōbìxuānquán*).

Somehow the Tai Chi Chuan characters have been interpreted in the West to mean only Supreme Ultimate Fist. Because the Tai Chi has been referred to as the Supreme Ultimate Goal, the translations have been confused over time. If Tai Chi is only seen as a martial art, it is difficult to understand the true meaning of the characters and catch the Li or function of the practice. The Martial Arts view can obscure the Li (function and essence) of Tai Chi as a path towards cultivation of the original self.

By balancing the dualism of Tai Chi in our body and our mind, the actions of dualism come to the front of our consciousness.
Tai Chi is, therefore, a method of recognizing dualism and opens the path for the ultimate return to non-dualism, or the Wu Chi. Chuan is to roll up ones sleeve and get to work earnestly to make that happen as an act of devotion or obeisance.

This balanced awareness that comes from practicing Tai Chi creates A Person who is able to be a "Centered Person Between Heaven and Earth Who Knows How to Stand Like a Tree, be Relaxed as a Pine Tree and Uses the Hand and the Mouth in a Balanced Fashion." This accomplishment leads to a clear and different way of being.

In order for true seeing to become a reality, there must be an alignment with the original Li source. Tai Chi provides that alignment. When this happens, the power of that original source comes forth into our awareness, a power that the ancient Chinese called Te (pronounced DUH).

One final note about the universal importance of the concept of Tai Chi can be found in the crest of Niels Bohr, the Nobel Peace price winner and great contributor to Quantum Mechanics and Atomic Structure. His personal crest contains the Tai Chi symbol and the Latin words: *contraria sunt complementa* or "opposites are complementary." What a reminder from a leader of 20 th century science!

Finally, your ultimate goal in taijiquan practice is to harmonize your energy with the energy of the natural universe. In order to achieve this goal, you must regulate your spirit (tiao shen, 調神) to a firm, strong, peaceful and enlightened state. Only then may you reach the final cultivation of the Dao: the unification of heaven (i.e., universe) and humanity (tian ren he yi, 天人合一). When you reach this stage, you will find that even your purpose in studying taijiquan, the very ego that holds the desire to learn and improve, will itself dissolve into the patterns of taiji.

Taijiquan is only the way or path to understanding life and comprehending the universe. As you near your goal, you will find that your motivation to learn martial arts is sublimated, and the health of your body, mind, and spirit can be unified and maintained without conscious effort."

Dr. Yang, Jwing-Ming

June 06, 2011

61

Richard Leirer

Chapter Four

Te or De

The Power Of Virtue and
The Energy To Do The Right Thing

As a result of Qigong/Tai Chi practice, I have become a more gentle, loving, stronger, yet softer man. One reason for this change is the development of the power of virtue, or Te, in my life that came about as a result of my practice. Te is a Chinese Character that can be translated as virtue. Sometimes it is also translated as power. I like to translate it as the power of virtue. Fung Yu Lan writes:

> According to Lao Tzu, Tao is that by which all things come to be. In this process of coming to be, each individual thing obtains something from the universal Tao, and this something is called Te...The Te of a

thing is what it naturally is.

(Yu-lan v.1 p.100).

The Li, or principle of everything, is also what it naturally is. Li and Te are linked. Te is the natural virtue, power or even grace that is embodied within all things. It lies with the Li or function of all things.

Te is the power that appears after finding the Li or function of a natural and balanced life.

The image for Te is made up of a number of separate images.

1) The image to the left of the ideogram describes two people.

2) The top cross on the image of Te represents the number 10 , a cross or a meeting place. It looks like this.

3) The sideways rectangular image below the cross represent the eyes, turned sideways.

The straight line underneath represents one.

4) The bottom characters means xin, or heart-mind.

One explanation for this ideogram is that the two people represent our two minds, the conditioned mind and our original mind. The top cross represents the cross above the eyes, or the third eye area. When the third eye area is activated, this area will allow us to experience the equanimity of all existence. The one stands for the one unity with the Tao and the original Li. The ability to think or have consciousness comes from our heart in Chinese Culture. The heart is the seat of consciousness in Chinese thought, not the brain. The heart is also the seat of our shen, soul or spirit.

The ancients believed a person has three types of spirit or consciousness or thinking, each is called shen (xin). There is the body xin, the Qi or energy xin, and the Tao xin, or the oneness of consciousness with all. The heart, the consciousness of the body contains both our wisdom mind and our emotional responses to external stimuli. The wisdom mind is known to be strong like a horse. The emotional mind is sometimes called the monkey mind. The heart consciousness of our Tao or Wu Chi existence is called our wisdom mind. Tao heart is our spiritual heart free from emotional encumbrances.

In other words when the third eye area is opened our heart will also open. With an open heart we will know Tao, as well as our true, original function (Li), and possibly the Wu Chi state.

Lao Tzu reminds us that, "He who does not deviate from the invariable Te, returns to the Limitless… He who has a sufficiency of the invariable Te, returns to a state of Unwrought Simplicity." TTC Ch 28 (Fung v.1 p.181)

This unwrought simplicity is our original mind and nature. Nature means what is spontaneous, so that, "To act by means of non-activity (wu wei) is called Nature… What is of Nature is internal. What is of man is external… That oxen and horses should have four feet is what is of Nature. That a halter should be put on a horse's head, or a string through an ox's nose, is what is of man." (Fung Yulan v.1 p.224)

 A real human being is said to be a person who has access to both minds and uses them appropriately according to each individual circumstance. A person who understands Te is a follower of the original consciousness and is often considered a sage.

A Qigong/Tai Chi person is asked to live according to the rightness of the moment. That rightness is a found in the Chinese expression " Feng Liu." Literally translated, it means, "wind and stream." Here is a story about a person who lives "Feng Liu" acting " according to Li, not according to others." This person is a person who follows his or her own original nature.

> A wise man woke up one day and had the thought to
> visit his friend who lived up river. It was a cold, windy
> and rainy day and he would need to travel up river
> in his boat by hand paddle to visit him. Having this
> thought in his mind, the wise man set out on his journey
> after breakfast. It took most of the day to complete his

journey. In the cold, wind and rain he finally arrives at his friend's house. The wise man secures his simple boat and begins to walk to his friend's front door. As he is walking to his friends front door, the wise man realized he no longer was thinking of his friend. The thought of his friend was no longer compelling him forward. Recognizing this, he returns to his boat and slowly returns home.

Never having completed his visit, he was still satisfied. The thought of his friend was no longer in his mind. The wise man honors the impulse and acts according to the circumstance directed by his true original mind. His own inner directions satisfy him. How many of us today would have to go through with the visit to our friend, simply because of all the trouble we went through? The conditioned mind says of course you finish and visit. The unconditioned original mind is content with the journey the natural impulse brings.

The one who follows the unconditioned mind, the original mind, or the inherent Te, is one who has faith in him/her self and has found the original Li. That faith is in the basic goodness that lies within each person. Flowing with the stream, each individual has present time access, which frees the conditioned "Shoulds" of our lives. My Tai Chi teacher Lee Henn, used to wear a tee shirt that said "Don't should on me." This teacher was living Feng Lui and encouraging others to do the same by wearing the shirt. By not "shoulding" on ourselves or others, we can begin to act naturally, according to each circumstance.

We then learn to rely on a basic goodness that is inherent in each moment of life and to honor our ability to access that goodness.

How do we know whether the wise man needed the experience of visiting his friend, or the experience that occurred while following his thoughts? Is it the ride or the destination that is important? The goal of the wise man was to follow his inner nature and not his outer programmed one.

The far-reaching extent of mental programming cannot be overstated. Current behavioral psychological thought attests to the depth of this programming, which prevents us from accessing the natural inherent Te, or power of the universe.

The great psychologist Carl Jung wrote a preface to an early translation of a Qigong Chinese text referred to as *The Secret of the Golden Flower.* This ancient text describes an alchemical process that was called "turning the light around" as a way to the awakening of the human potential. Jung hoped we all could awaken to the potential that lies hidden within most of us. In his personal writings, he speaks of being inspired by Chinese philosophy, particularly the *I Ching*. The *I Ching*, is the first known-recorded discussion of the Tai Chi idea.

Qigong /Tai Chi then, is an ancient concept that has at its root individual transpersonal growth. This is accomplished by breaking away from conditioned thought and through an awakening to each individual's human and spiritual potential. Practical methods of transpersonal growth that have been refined over the ages can be easily learned and eventually mastered with continuous practice and application.

Jung says in his commentary on *The Secret of the Golden Flower*:

> If the unconscious can be recognized as a co-determining quantity along with the conscious, and if we can live in such a way that conscious and unconscious, or instinctive demands, are given recognition as far as possible, the center of gravity of the total personality shifts its position. It ceases to be in the ego, which is merely the centre of

consciousness, and instead is located in a hypothetical point between the conscious and the unconscious, which might be called the true self. (Wilhelm p.124)

Awakening to this other mind cannot overcome all of the programming that has been accumulated over time. The famous master Kuei-Shan Ling-Yu (771-853 A.D.) explains saying:

> Does a person who has sudden awakening still need to continue with cultivation? If one has true awakening and attains the fundamental, then at that time that person knows for himself that cultivation and non cultivation are just dualistic opposites. Like now, though the initial inspiration is dependent on conditions, if within a single thought one awakens to one's own reality, there are still habitual tendencies that have accumulated over numberless kalpas which cannot be purified in a single instant. That person should certainly be taught how to gradually remove the karmic tendencies and mental habits: This is cultivation, there is no other method of cultivation that needs to be taught to that person. (Cheng Chen Bhikshu p.25)

What, then, is cultivation of Te? It is the work needed to realize what is not realized. This is the "Gong" part of Qigong. Gong means to cultivate, work with, turn over, and practice.

What type of practice and cultivation is needed for this awakened transformation to happen?

First, one must cultivate the skill of awareness followed by the cultivation of the Qi or life energy and finally connection with the power of Te. Through this cultivation a person can find the original self and original Li. Only the cultivated person has awakened to the Te, the virtue, and the universal power.

How a person can cultivate life energy, awaken the unconditioned mind and overcome the programmed mental tendencies that may have accumulated over numberless lifetimes of existence is the primary focus of this book. These chapters are designed to help awaken the concept of another level of being and thinking beyond the average conditioned mind thinking and give practical Qigong and Tai Chi movements to practice.

An ancient Chinese sage Chang Po-Tuan clearly describes this mental relationship in Thomas Cleary's translated *"The Inner Teachings of*

Taoism." Master Po did not begin his cultivation until his mid 60's. He wrote his great work on "Cultivating Reality" in his 90's. He says:

> Our conditioned knowledge has the Yin energy of earth like the fullness that is in the triagram for water. Our unconditioned mind has the Yang energy from heaven and is represented by the triagram for fire. The great alchemical change can occur if an individual takes the unconditioned information and becomes aware of it consciously.

Kan   Water

Li Fire

This is known as the union of Kan and Li, or the merging of Fire and Water. It is also known as "when the light of the two eyes become one," or as the Sun and Moon containing the vitality of reality. This is the secret of the Golden Flower. If one can understand that these two energies belong to one another, then one can cultivate backwards. Cultivating backwards means using the body to find the Qi, using the Qi to find the shen or spirit, and using the spirit to return to the Wu Chi. Master Po:

> Inverting water and fire, using real knowledge to control conscious knowledge, using conscious knowledge to nurture real knowledge, water and fire balance each other, movement and stillness are as one; then mind is Tao, Tao is mind. Mind is the mind of Tao, body is the body of Tao, sharing the qualities of heaven and earth, sharing the light of the sun and moon, sharing the order of the seasons – the whole world is within one's own body. (Cleary p.25)

What happens as a result of this merging of fire and water is an awakening of the real human in connection with the Li and Te of life. The essence of each individual does not exist only within the human body as a part of a permanent condition. We are all also spirit. We are all part of the Wu Chi. We have existed before we have existed in form. Our real mind or

74

consciousness is not in the human brain. It is beyond that limited human view and includes an awareness of the cosmos free from form. ThisSuper Consciousness is outside of the human brain. However, the brain is the controller of the body and the area where information is encoded. Your real mind is the controller of the brain. Your real mind is the operator of that great human computer called the brain. An individual who has awakened to this reality is said to have produced this spiritual embryo. This is the realization of the spiritual self. This spiritual self is freed from the constraints of the body as evidenced by those who have had near death experiences or out of body experiences.

Many who have experienced this state can experience the world outside of the body. The out of body experience is a real one. It can be acquired through practice and training. That training involves a reversal, a going back to the time first of the child, then the infant, and finally the embryo. Going beyond the mbryo, a person then can discover their original face or original nature before conception. A commonality in many spiritual traditions is the idea that one must become like a child.

In Qigong/Tai Chi, this means reawakening the original mind that existed before birth, was strong as a child, and whole as an embryo. Master Kuei -Shan Ling-Yu reminds us that even after we awaken to this idea, there

Richard Leirer

is still cultivation to do. It is the complete return to our original mind. Again Master Chang Po-Tuan reminds us.

> Before one's parents give birth to one's body, when the yin and yang energies of male and female interact, in the midst of darkness there is a point of living potential, which comes forth from nothing. This is called the primordial, true, unified generative energy. This energy enters the sperm and ovum, fusing them into one: formless, it produces form; immaterial, it produces substance. At this point. though there is the human form, there is no human way; nothing in the world, not even water, fire, or weapons, can harm one here. (Cleary p.60 – 61)

The ultimate goal in our practice is to return to this state, through observation, meditation, awareness, and energy circulation of Tai Chi/ Qigong.

Observation has shown that after ten months the embryo is born as an infant. The sages say at our birth, this is what we experienced:

at the moment of that cry, the conscious spirit of the generations of history also enters into the opening and merges with the primordial original spirit. The original spirit depends on the conscious spirit to subsist, while the conscious spirit depends on the original spirit for effective awareness. (Cleary p.62)

This is the same concept as the Jungian collective unconscious. This idea that "the conscious spirits of the generations of history" can enter into each individual consciousness is part of Chinese philosophy.

Here as an infant the original energy and original mind is still in charge. The conditioned mind has not yet taken over. Soon the infant grows into a child. The child begins to discriminate and gain cognition. Master Po clearly tells us:

Though there is discrimination and cognition, the encrustation of the faculties has not yet taken place and acquired influences have not yet invaded; when hungry, one eats, and when cold, one just puts on clothes. Joy, anger, sadness, and happiness come and go, vanishing as they arise; one does not know about differences of wealth and status, but is

spontaneous and has no extraneous thoughts. This,

too, is the germ and embryo of sages, the root and

sprout of immortals and Buddha's....They both

(child and infant) are imbued with natural reality,

but they are different in terms of state, the infant

being higher and the child lower. (Cleary p.63)

So as a child, we can be like a sage. The child, infant, and embryo
are in harmony with the environment of Te. This is when most of us
were the happiest. The level of consciousness is great, and there is no
imbalance in the elements in the body. The organs and acupuncture
channels are in balance.

However, as the child grows into maturity,

discriminatory awareness gradually arises, and the

encrustation's of the senses gradually takes place;

the real retreats and the artificial assumes authority.

Now even the state of the Child is lost. (Cleary p.65)

The individual is now filled with the conditioned mind or the mind of man. The original mind, the mind of Tao has been forgotten. The way of the sage is lost. Imbalance appears in the elements; the acupuncture channels go awry. Harmony is lost and the road to destruction is set in motion. In short, the pursuit of desires of the conditioned thinking sends the individual into a downward decline. Our celestial energy gradually wanes. The life force cannot be sustained and death is inevitable.

In Qigong and Tai Chi, we want to restore the original energy and our awareness of the original mind and open to the power of Te. Following the inner guide within ourselves, we can return to our original nature and access power and virtue from that place. Practice is the way of finding that glorious, wonderful, inner nature that yearns to be free. Qigong and Tai Chi practice connects us to the universal Tao. All our talents that have been hidden under the conditioned thinking are waiting to be uncovered.

Imagine the contributions to the world that will be lost if those talents are not released? As the return takes place, joy and happiness fill the world. A lost child has now been found. The prodigal child has returned. The world will rejoice if even one person awakens, for finding the way is of benefit to all humankind. When one child returns, the collective unconscious in us all is empowered. Each of us knows we have the same potential. Those gifts we will bring will change the world.

Trust in yourself and in the power of what attracted you to these words. You know if they ring true.

The course of returning through Qigong/Tai Chi is one of many paths a person could follow. For whatever reason you have been drawn to this path or teaching. In my opinion, there is a path similar in thought to the Qigong/Tai Chi way that was formed in the United States. It is called *A Course in Miracles* and is published by the Foundation For Inner Peace. The introduction to the course states,

> This is a course in miracles. It is a required course. Only the time you take it is voluntary…. The course does not aim at teaching the meaning of love, for that is beyond what can be taught. It does aim however, at removing the blocks to the awareness of love's presence, which is your natural inheritance… This course can therefore be summed up very simply in this way: 'Nothing real can be threatened. Nothing unreal exists. Herein lies the peace of God. *A Course in Miracles Volume One: Text.*

This is the same goal in Qigong/Tai Chi, to remove the blocks to the awareness of not only Love's presence, but also the blocks to our own existence. Removing the blocks frees us all to our relationship with God, the Tao, the enlightened consciousness, the Wu Chi. When these blocks are removed, we will have discovered who we are.

Marianne Williamson, teacher of the Course in Miracles aptly states:

Our deepest fear is not that we are inadequate. Our deepest fear is that we are powerful beyond measure. It is our light, not our darkness that most frightens us. We ask ourselves, Who am I to be brilliant, gorgeous, talented and fabulous? Actually, who are we not to be? You are a child of God. Your playing small doesn't serve the world. There's nothing enlightened about shrinking so that other people won't feel insecure around you. We were born to make manifest the glory of God that is within us. It is not just in some of us; it's in everyone. And as we let our own light shine, we unconsciously give other people permission to do the same. As we are liberated from our own fear, our presence automatically liberates others. (Williamson

p.190-191)

The goal in *The Course In Miracles* is to use your thoughts to awaken to love's presence. In Qigong/Tai Chi, the goal is to use the energy to remove the obstacles to your true self. The circulation of the energy through the acupuncture channels will have a certain effect. One will be a removal of the blockages in the channels, which erases the conditioned thinking.

In Qigong/Tai Chi, if the energy blockages are removed, the individual will naturally return the original state. No need to use thought to get there. In fact, I believe it is much more difficult to use thought to change the way I think and perceive the world around me than it is to do some simple energy exercises. By doing the exercises, the conditioned thinking is released, and the individual awakens to the unconditioned true self. The thought process changes by awakening to the real mind that is within each of us.

Just run the energy and watch what will happen. Like running a magnet over a computer disc, the information stored in the computer disc will be erased. Running energy through the body can also erase our conditioned mind. The running of the energy in the acupuncture channels, particularly the Ren Mai and Tu Mai channels is the key component in the reversal process and erasing process. Opening all of the eight special channels begins with these front and back channels. What is this energy that can erase that programmed conditioning? The ancient Chinese masters called it Qi (Chi).

When this Qi or life energy is able to circulate freely and naturally within the body, old patterns of thinking fall away. The blockage of this energy can come from blocking the original self. The more the original self is blocked, the more restricted the Li and the Te of the original self, creating less Qi flow. Indian gurus as well as Chinese sages discovered the same truths.

From the spiritual teachings of Ramana Maharshi we hear this.

> Truly there is no cause for you to be miserable and unhappy. You yourself impose limitations on your true nature of infinite Being, and then weep that you are a finite creature. Hence I say know that you are really the infinite, pure Being, the self absolute. You are always that self and nothing but that Self.

Therefore, you can never really be ignorant of the Self; your Ignorance is merely a formal Ignorance. (Maharshi p.92)

The Chinese sage Po Tu-An expresses the same principle.

Ch'eng Hao says man's original state is that of union with the universe which, however becomes lost through the assertion of the individual ego... That which at birth is called the nature. The tendency toward life of all things is what is most worthy of our observation. What is great and originating becomes (in man) the first and Chief (quality of goodness). This quality is known as love (jen). Love is something that makes for oneness with Heaven and Earth...The man of love takes Heaven, Earth and all things as one with himself. To him there is nothing that is not himself...Thus if the hand or foot lack love, the vital force (Chi) will fail to circulate through them, and thus things will not be integrated with the self...The student must first comprehend love (jen). The man of love is undifferentiably one with other things...Get to comprehend this truth and cultivate it with sincerity (ch'eng) and earnestness (Ching); that is all. There is no need to impose any other rules or pursue any other search. (Fung Yu-Lan v2 p.520, 521)

Richard Leirer

Chapter Five

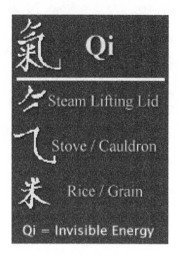

Qi or Chi
The Life Force Of The Universe And The Engine Of Our Body.

The mystery of Qi (pronounced Chi) is at the center of Chinese Traditional Medicine and the cornerstone of the Qigong/Tai Chi practice. It is the key to cultivation and the secret to finding the original self. I thought I knew what Qi was early in my martial arts training because I could break a board or brick with a punch or a kick. Later I thought I knew what Qi was when I felt my hands being tingly or hot after my Qigong or Tai Chi practice. It was only after working with Master Hao Tien You that I really did catch the feeling of the Qi and become able to circulate and control it. Thank you Master Hao for all that you taught me and for having patience with me in my training. He often said to me "If you don't move the Qi when doing Tai Chi and Qigong, you might as well go disco, you will get better benefit."

Qi is said to be a vital energy that exists as a physical reality. In the human body, at conception, we were given a certain amount of Qi (sometimes called Yuan Qi or Jing) from our parents. "This Qi is partly responsible for an individual's inherited constitution. It is stored in the Kidneys. " (Kaptchuk p.36)

When an individual's original Qi is gone, his /her human life will no longer exist. This prenatal energy is a finite, limited quantity. The more we preserve this Qi, the longer we will live.

To preserve this energy the body supplements its original Qi with Qi from breath (kong-Qi) and Qi from food (gu-Qi). As a person brings this postnatal Qi into the body thru eating and breathing, the body uses this energy to perform action.

Movement, metabolism, and even thinking require energy or Qi. The normal process of using energy for life activities puts oneself in a deficit situation. More expenditure of Qi and fewer savings of Qi lead to a loss of Qi, particularly our original jing Qi. Most of us use more postnatal Qi in the course of a day then what we bring into the body, putting us in a deficit situation with Qi. More energy is used, and not enough energy is brought into the body thru normal activities to equal the normal expenditure of energy. With this deficit condition, a withdrawal must be made from the original energy (Jing) and a depletion of the original energy occurs.

A normal lifetime simply allows the body to slowly decline (age). This usage of original energy occurs because the individual is performing action and the body needs energy to accomplish that action. If the input of energy does not equal the output of energy the body must pull more energy from the Jing Qi that is stored in the kidneys. The normal functions of eating food and breathing generally do not supply enough sources of energy to stop the withdrawal of energy from the Jing or original energy storehouse. The continued withdrawing of this original energy occurs and death is the result of using up all the Qi.

Master Hao told me that the average person is given enough original energy to last five times the number of years needed to grow the permanent molars or wisdom teeth. These teeth typically come in during our late teens or early 20's. The average, healthy life span for most people is about 100 to 120 years.

The goal in our practice is to concentrate and increase the postnatal Qi of food and breath. If Qi could be concentrated and developed inside the body then aging would decline and health would always be maintained. This is the premise of health. Qi energy in sufficient amounts nourishes the body. Eating properly and storing the Qi from breathing are two most important concepts in Qigong Tai Chi practice. This way, less energy is withdrawn from the original energy (Jing), and the postnatal energy (food and breath) is adequate to equal the energy needed to get through a day. No loss of Jing, no loss of life. Less loss of Jing Qi, longer life span.

One of the easiest way to increase Qi, and therefore our longevity, is to practice this technique: Breath in, think of the chest area, feel the Qi you just breathed in, breath out move the Qi with your mind down to the Xia Dan Tian, or lower abdomen. This exercise directs the Qi entering the body from breath, and it also takes the Qi that remains from food that is in your stomach and intestines and stores the residual in the Xia Dan Tien. This technique is called *Qi Chen Xia Dan Tien* or referred to as the opening of the ren acupuncture channel pass.

The Famous Tai Chi master Yue Tan mentions in his work, *The Principles of Tai Chi,*

'Practice to Turn Jing into Qi' as primary. it demands that Zhong Qi should be raised to the point Shanzhong, that situates at the center of the two nipples, and it should never exceed the point of quepen when one breathes in, or he may feel flushed and short of breath. And it demands that Zhong Qi should be lowered to Dantian when one breathes out. This is what the saying means: 'letting the acquired Qi direct the inborn Qi and then letting the latter transform the former.'

He further comments on the deficit situation we have when we use our prenatal Qi. Reminding us this situation can be addressed, he states the following.

Anyone who intends to change such a condition of ever growing deficit must break through Ren channel so as to have Zhong Qi to be conditioned to go downward, and thus one will be provided with the basic condition for rejuvenation. (ibid p 43)

With Qi in the body, it becomes a physical entity with physical parameters working within the human body. The body then uses the Qi energy in specific ways which is evident in the five types of Qi that are most important for the human body's functioning. These five types of Qi are explained by Ted Kaptchuk, in *The Web That Has No Weaver*, his guide to understanding Chinese Medicine.

"**Organ Qi** – Every organ is conceived as having its own Qi, whose activity is characterized by the organ to which it is attached.

Meridian Qi – The energy pathways through which Qi flow among the Organs and the various bodily parts, adjusting and harmonizing their activity. Each organ has a corresponding pathway or meridian the Qi flows along. Those pathways are called meridians.

Nutritive Qi – This Qi manifests itself in the Blood and moves with the blood through the Blood Vessels.

Protective Qi – This is the Qi responsible for resisting and combating Eternal Pernicious Influences (germs, virus, etc) when they invade the body. This Qi protects us from outside influences.

Ancestral Qi – Its main function is to aid and regulate the rhythmic movements of respiration and heartbeat, and so it is intimately connected with the Lungs and Heart." (Kaptchuk p.36)

Meridian Qi encompasses the Acupuncture lines or Qi channels that are the rivers the Qi flows through in the human body. Most of the acupuncture lines are specifically related to particular organs. There are important supplementary channels that exist as well. However, it can be said that there are a basic 20 channels in the human body. Twelve of these are related to an internal organ and its function. Eight others are known as special extraordinary channels not related to a particular organ. These eight channels are also called the physic channels.

There are also numerous collateral channels linking the Qi to every cell and part of the physical body.

The most important of these 20 channels are the Ren channel that runs in front of the body and the Tu channel that runs along the back of the body. The back channel feeds and nourishes all of the yang organs and acupuncture channels in the body, and the front Ren channel feeds and nourishes all of the Yin channels and Yin organs. The abundance of energy in these two channels and the free circulation of energy are the first important goals of the Qigong/Tai Chi practitioner and are known as the small heavenly circulation or the microcosmic orbit (*Xiao Zhou Tian*).

The very famous empty force Tai Chi master Yue Huanzhi tells us that the way to practice Tai Chi is through stages.

> Generally, it may be said in this way: learn to practice a whole set of Taijiquan first and do it with care, he may find it beneficial to both the body and the mind and then he should ask some well-known Qigong masters to instruct him some simple and easy Qigong…try to learn the ropes of the internal Gonfu and taste carefully its savour, he may be considered to have completed the primary school if he can, through constant practice, be patient to break through Ren Channel and come up to the level of " Practicing to Turn Jing into Qi." The second stage is that one must add Qigong to the practice of Taijiquan-doing. To be more concrete, he must try hard to make Ren and Du channels passable to form Xiao Zhou Tian… (Yue Tan p. 5).

The Xiao Xhou Tian is the circulation of Qi through the Ren and Du channels that most effects health in the human body. If a person can get the Qi to pass through the tail bone into the back Tu channel, and then to lead the Qi up the back to the top of the head, this is half of the heavenly circulation. The Du channel travels over the top of the head and stops at the upper lip, under the nose. The Ren channel Qi travels down the front of the body, connecting with the Du channel when the tip of the tongue touches the roof of the mouth. It then meets the Du channel again at the bottom of the trunk, the perineum or *hui yin* acupuncture point. If the Qi can circulate through these channels in a continuous fashion, health will ensue. Trauma from the birth process, (being born), blocked the Du channel at the tailbone (*wei lu*) lower back (*ming men*), mid back (*tao tao*), neck (*da jui*) and base of the brain (*yue ren*). In order for the energy to pass through this back channel a person must have an abundance of Qi energy stored in the lower Xia Dantian. This is a storage place located below the navel. With an abundance of energy at this location a person will have enough power and Qi to break through the areas along the Du channel.

Practicing sending Qi down from the chest (*Qi chen xia dan tien*) will open the Ren channel on the front of the trunk, and get Qi trained to flow down to the Dan Tien for storage. The blockage of the Ren channel usually takes place at the solar plexus or stomach area. Breaking through the blockages is a key to health and awakening. This step is known as "Practicing to turn Jin into Qi" or *Lien Jing Hwa Qi*.

When this energy can be freely circulated up and down the body, a remarkable event occurs. The conditioned thinking accumulated within can be erased. It is as if this energy moving through the body is acting like a magnet that is erasing the information stored on a computer hard drive of our body. It is said that if the energy can be circled one million times, an evolutionary change will occur in the body. Roy Eugene Davis, a key disciple of the great Indian mystic Paramahansa Yogananda explains.

> Theoretically, if a person could inhabit a body for one million years, under natural, healthful conditions, due to this tendency for refinement, at the end of this time there would be a refinement of brain tissue which would be suitable for the manifestation of cosmic consciousness. (Davis p.181)

Paramahansa Yogananda taught the practice of Kriya Yoga. This is a type of yoga that also circulates the Qi or prana energy up the back channel, and down the front channel in a similar fashion to the Qigong practiced just mentioned. Davis and my masters have said that if a person runs the small heaven one million times, that person would evolve into a new human being. A real human being, freed from the programmed conditioning and following his Li direct from the universe, uniting with the universal Te or virtue.

This new person would be flowing with the Tao, inwardly directed, and in living life in a sacred manner. The circulation of Qi energy through the Tu and Ren channels can speed an individual's personal evolution.

To accomplish this circulation, it is important to find the feeling of the Qi and use the Qi to open the paths. Knowing Qi is real, and can be felt or perceived through the sense of touch and feeling, is a key element of practice. The use of imagination is a hindrance in discovering the feeling of the Qi. This feeling is vital for the proper circulation and direction of Qi, by the mind and is an essential stage in our cultivation.

Some key research here in the United States indicated, "acupuncture meridians have transmission like characteristics" (Reichmanis, M IEEE *Transactions of Biomedical Electronics* 22 (1975) 553 & (1977): 402.)

Understanding Qi as a medium that travels through channels and not an imaginary force will go a long way in training.

The use of acupuncture to anesthetize certain areas of animals bodies has grown to have the American Veterinarian Association endorse acupuncture as a method for animal treatment, and is recommended for analgesic purposes.

Imagine convincing your dog Fido there is no pain when he is having surgery. Acupuncture works on the basis of Qi and the properties it manifest through each channel. Qigong/Tai Chi is acupuncture without needles. Qigong/Tai Chi is the ability to circulate the Qi energy throughout all the acupuncture channels in the human body by the power of the mind. No need to use a needle.

Of the hundreds of research papers written in China over the years on Qi, what is becoming apparent is that Qi can be measured and does have an effect at a distance. However Qi seems to behave differently based on the method of observation. Whatever its physical properties, what is apparent is the effects. If the Qi circulates in harmony in the body, health is abundant. Mental habits disappear and original thinking becomes dominant.

As for the question of what is Qi, see the work of Gu Hansen who reported work on qi in 1979 from the Shanghai Institute of Atomic Research. She concluded that external Qi was and is a measurable physical substance and a form of "particle current."

Further experiments in collaboration with the Shanghai Institute of Chinese Medicine concluded, "the qigong practitioner emitted electromagnetic waves containing information." In 1979 the research team presented a demonstration of the experiments to the directors of the State Science Commission, The National Association for Science and Technology (NAST), the Ministry of Health and the State Sports Commission. The report claimed 'qi has a materiel basis and objectively exists', and described seven types of physical manifestations of qi. (Paper p.53)

Taiji is actually the motive force generated from the mind (Yi). From this force, the Qi is led and circulates throughout the body. Summing up, Taijiquan is the martial style which trains the practitioner to use the mind to lead the Qi, circulating it in the body, and generating the Yin and Yang states, either for health, fighting, or otherwise.

Dr. Yang, Jwing-Ming June 23 2009

Chapter Six

Tzu Ran or Ziran

What Is Natural: The Way To Align With Our True Nature

Tzu Ran is an image that represents the natural Li power that comes forth from the Tao. This image is complex and combines the ideograms for self, great, fire and an idea or state of being that is natural or spontaneous within itself. Tzu Ran is the natural expression of Li. The power of Te can only issue forth if there is a following of Tzu Ran or what is natural.

Lao Tzu says,

Man follows the Earth

Earth follows Heaven

Heaven follows Tao

Tao follows what is natural. (Tzu Ran)

(Chapter 25 of the Tao Te Ching: Gia

– Fu Feng Translation)

The first character Tzu 自 is the character for self. The self is composed of a combination of sun (Ri 日) and moon (yue 月).

So a person is composed of the energy of the sun and the moon. In Neigong Qigong practice this is known as the right and left eye. The energy of those eyes becomes focused into a single point during meditation. In Christian terminology Jesus said in Matthew 6:22-23 "The light of the body is the eye: if therefore thine eye be single, thy whole body shall be full of light." In the Gospel of Thomas 22, Jesus says, "When you make the two one, and when you make the inside as the outside, and the outside as the inside, and the upper as the lower, and when you make the male and the female into a single one, so that the male is not male and the female not female, and when you make eyes in place of an eye, and a hand in place of a hand, and a foot in place of a foot, an image in place of an image, then shall you enter (the kingdom). (*Gospel of Thomas Saying 22 earlychristianwritings.com.*

n.p., n.d. web nov 2012)

The second character in Tzu Ran is the character for correct or right,

Ran 然.

Ziran is also a compound character for self, fire and heart. This is a condition when the light of the two eyes becomes one within the self in order to have correct action. In Buddhism it is called right action and leads to right livelihood.

Tzu Ran, in Chinese philosophy is expressed by the previously mentioned story about a person who lives "according to himself" but not according to others. The story is about a wise man, who woke up one day and had the thought to visit his friend who lived up the river.

 The wise man honors the impulse and acts according to the circumstance directed by his own mind. His own inner directions satisfy him and he disregards the ramblings of others. He listens to his true self, deciding how to live, what to do.

Chuang-tzu says,

The people have a constant nature: to weave and clothe themselves, till and feed themselves. This is the common nature of all, and everyone agrees with it. This is said to be sent by Nature (Tzu Ran). And so in the age when the nature of man was perfect, men moved quietly and gazed steadfastly. At that time, there were no roads over the mountains or boats and bridges to cross the water. Things were born and matured, each attached to its own native locality. Birds and beasts multiplied; trees and shrubs grew up. The former could be led by the hand. One could climb and peep into the raven's nest. In this age of perfect nature, men dwelt together with birds and beasts, and the human race was one with all things. How could there be knowledge of the distinctions of superior and inferior men? All being equally without knowledge, their instincts (te) did not leave them. All being equally lacking in desires, they may be said to have been in a state of Unadorned Simplicity (su p'u). Being in this state, they had possession of their original natures. (Tzu Ran) (Fung Yulan v.1 p.227)

In another example of following Tzu Ran, from another story related in the Chuang-tzu,

> Of old, when a seabird alighted outside the capital of Lu, the Marquis of Lu went out to receive it, gave it wine in the temple, and had the Chiu Shao music played to amuse it, and a bullock slaughtered to feed it. But the bird was dazed and too timid to eat or drink anything. In three days it was dead. This was treating the bird as one would treat oneself, and not as a bird would treat a bird. Had he treated it as a bird would have treated a bird, he would have put it to roost in a deep forest, allowed it to wander over the plain, to swim in a river or lake, to feed upon fish, to fly in formation (with others), and to settle leisurely. When it already hated hearing human voices, fancy adding music! Play the Hsien Ch'ih and Chiu Shao in the wilds of Tung-t'ing, and on hearing it birds will fly off, beasts will run away, and fish will dive below. But men will gather together to listen.
>
> (Fung Yulan v.1 p.228)

Don't we all want to please our parents, our teachers, our husbands, wives and lovers? How many of us treat ourselves, as we need to be treated, and not how others want us to be? If we let others treat us in a manner that is not of our true nature we will die inside. As in the above story, in three days our Qi will stop flowing. Our natural life cycle will be cut short all because we let others treat us as they want to see us, and not treat us as we truly are. Worse still is how we treat ourselves and the way we hinder our original true nature.

Shen Tao, a Chinese Sage says,

> When birds fly in the air and fish swim in the deeps,
> they do not do so through any conscious art. Therefore
> birds and fish do not, themselves, know that they are
> capable of flying and swimming; if they knew this, and
> set their minds on doing it, they would inevitably fall
> down and be drowned. It is likewise with the moving
> of a man's feet and grasping of his hands, the listening
> of his ears, and seeing of his eyes. At the same time
> of their moving, grasping, hearing, and seeing, these
> act so of their own accord at the proper occasion, and

do not wait for the act of thinking before doing so. If they had to wait for thought before acting, they would become exhausted. Hence, it is those persons who accord themselves with the spontaneous (tzu jan) who long survive, and those who attain to the constant norm who win out. (Fung Yulan v.1 p.155)

This is our goal: To live and be who we naturally are, and not live as others want us to be. Some of us have been taught that we are essentially not good, and many have been told they are indeed naturally bad. Some believe we have to be taught to be good as if goodness were something outside of the self and must be taught. An ancient Chinese story tells of a person who hears the cries of a child who fell into a well. How would a person respond naturally to this situation?

What is the root of good and evil? Must we be trained to be good? If everyone did what they wanted, would there be chaos and anarchy? Master Wang says no.

Master Wang explained:

The highest good is the mind's original substance.

Whatever goes beyond this original substance (Tzu Ran) is evil. It is not the case of there being something good, and then of there being something evil standing in opposition to it. Thus being good and evil are only a single thing.

When I heard this statement by the master, I understood the saying of Master Ch'eng that goodness, to be sure, certainly belongs to the nature (Tzu Ran), yet evil cannot be said to belong also to nature. Good and evil are both Heavenly Principle. What we call evil is not original evil, but results either from transgressing or falling short of our original nature. (Tzu Ran). (Fung Yulan v.2 p.614)

Our original nature is good. It is what naturally and spontaneously flows from the Tao, from Heaven. It is our Tzu Ran. However, we can be taught to be evil. When we hear cries of a child that has fallen into a well, what is our original thought?

Our first thought is what is from heaven, that spontaneous action to save the child. Do we wait and think, "is that my enemy's child?" or "will I get sued?" Do we say, "there is nothing I can do," or "don't get involved?" No, all these thoughts come second and have been programmed into our minds. That is where the evil comes into our lives: it is taught.

Following Tzu Ran, what is natural for you in thoughts, words and deeds and what will come forth from within, will benefit the whole world.

When I was in my thirties and had been training in Qigong/Tai Chi and Wushu since I was eighteen, I had an experience of not following what was natural. I was at my friend Doug's wedding reception. His brother invited his friend who was a linebacker for Miami University, an Ohio college football team. He was about 6 ft, 4 in. tall and weighed over 220 lbs and was in great physical shape. I was 5 ft 8in about 140 lbs and full of martial arts confidence. Somehow our conversation turned to arm wrestling. Before long we were piling up phone books under my elbow so my hand could reach his, and we could begin our arm wrestling challenge. I told my arm not to move. I told my muscles to hold. They did. As we pushed into each other, straining to win I felt my arm being very strong. Then there was a very loud cracking sound. It filled the room and sounded like a gunshot.

Brian the football player, leaped back in his chair and we both looked in amazement as my arm floated to the right in an angle that everyone present knew was not right. I stared at my right arm laying flat on the table on the right side of my body. I did not feel any pain, yet I could not move that arm. I quietly asked if someone would please help me get my arm. It would not work and I could not reach it with my left hand, it was too far to the right of my body. Someone helped me retrieve my arm, and I stood up and started walking out the door when Doug's brother yelled, "Where are you going?" I said, "To the hospital. I just broke my arm." Of course he insisted on driving me, and sure enough, my arm was completed broken and shattered in the middle of the upper arm or humerus. My muscles did their job: they did not tear or rip or shatter. Normally, the muscle will tear first under the great strain and force in the arm wrestling contest. Instead, my arm snapped in two as a result of that force being applied by the muscles to the two edges of the bone.

My arm did not follow what was natural because my mind gave it an instruction to do something else. I demonstrated a lack of humility and a deep over-confidence in my training. I learned a great lesson in humility that day, and recognized a pattern within my own thinking that can lead to conflict and potential disharmony. I have a tendency to push beyond normal structure. Sometimes this is helpful, other times it is not.

Learning how to go with the natural flow is part of the benefit of Tai

Chi and Qigong training. Learning that arrogance can spring forth from conditioned thinking is taught by the Chinese story of the cricket who thought so much of himself that he stood in road in front of the horse drawn carriage and demanded that the carriage stop. SPLAT.

Chapter 51 of the Dao De Jing:

Through dao ten thousand things

have emerged and are alive.

Through de (virtue) they get fostered,

Through wu (thing-ing) they get configured,

Through Qi (instrumental doing) they

get completed and finished.

Therefore the ten thousand things

esteem dao and honor de (virtue).

Dao is esteemed and de is honored

without having merit.

They appropriate themselves as zi ran (it-self-so-ing).

Therefore, because of dao the ten thousand

things have emerged and are alive,

They are fostered,

They are growing, nurturing, maturing,

ripening, reserving and declining.

To keep alive without possession,

To act without holding on,

To grow without lording over,

This is called the profound de (virtue).

Translated by Prof. Qingjie James Wang

Chapter Seven

Tao or Dao
The Way And Path Of A Balanced Person

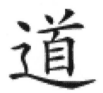

The above image for Tao is made up of a number of separate images.

1) The image on the left side of the Tao character is made up of the image for a path or road. Sometimes it is depicted as a person walking on a path or traveling on a journey.

2) The two top strokes of the image to the right of the character

represent yin and yang.

3) The next stroke is a horizontal line representing one.

一

4) The bottom rectangle with the two inner lines with the slash on top represents the ideogram for self. This is also composed of two separate ideograms for the sun 日 and the character for moon 月.

Combined, this creates the character for the self.

Tao is a description of how a person (self) can become one, through the balance of yin and yang energies, while traveling on a journey here on Earth. Tao is being in balance with all of who we are and what we can become, even as our Li, or function changes. Finding Tao is being able to constantly change in a balanced way. Becoming aligned with the Tao is our greatest struggle and can be our greatest achievement. Note: See Eva Wong's *Cultivating Stillness* p.12 for Tao image breakdown and meaning.)

In Qigong/Tai Chi practice being aligned with Tao is following the Tai

Chi Yin and Yang energies. Also following the Li principle of every moment and increasing awareness of Tzu Ran, what is natural at all times. That awareness comes through the practice of the merger of the energy from the right and left eye in Neigong Qigong practice. There is an old Quaker saying that says when the light of the two eyes becomes one, you will know God. This comes from the Book of Thomas mentioned earlier. Also, the first English translations of the word Tao, was God.

The ancient Chinese sage Chang Po-Tuan clearly describes this mental and energetic relationship:

> Inverting water and fire, using real knowledge to control conscious knowledge, using conscious knowledge to nurture real knowledge, water and fire balance each other, movement and stillness are as one; then mind is Tao, Tao is mind. Mind is the mind of Tao, body is the body of Tao, sharing the qualities of heaven and earth, sharing the light of the sun and moon, sharing the order of the seasons – the whole world is within one's own body. (Chang Po Tuan p.25)

This is Tao. To find our original mind that is one with the universe is our goal in cultivation. The path is through balance. That path includes the ability to speak in a balanced fashion, to nurture ourselves as we nurture others and be in touch with our original nature. Creating this relationship within ourselves and with the world around us is harmony. Thinking for our selves, living from our natural core while being aware of the relationship with the outside world is balance. With this balance our conditioned mind and our original mind can converse. Decisions can be made free from the influence of conditioning if we empower our original nature.

Manifesting an internal integrity that will never be taken away, we will be able to walk the earth in a balanced way.

Ch 55 of the *Tao Te Ching*

> One who embraces Tao
>
> Becomes pure and innocent
>
> Like a newborn babe
>
> Deadly insects will not sting him
>
> Wild beasts will not attack him
>
> Birds of prey will not strike him ...
>
> Things in harmony with the Tao remain

Things that are forced, grow for awhile

But then wither away

This is not keeping with Tao

Whatever is not keeping with Tao

Comes to an early end.

(Jonathan Star Translation)

It can take a while to awaken to new ideas and new insights that bring about harmony. In reading Oliver Sacks, I was taken by his "awakening" through observation of what appeared to be the illness of Tourette's appearing a thousand times more frequently in the general population than previously recorded.

He notes:

A very similar situation happened with muscular dystrophy, which was never seen until Duchenne described it in the 1850's. By 1860, after his original description, many hundreds of cases had been recognized and described, so much so that Charcot said: "How come that a disease so common, so widespread, and so recognizably

at a glance – a disease which has doubtless always
existed- how come that it is only recognized now?
.Why did we need M. Duchenne to open our eyes?

It is obvious that everyone was inattentionally blinded. How much more
are we blinded from seeing only what we want to see? Have we begun
to open our eyes collectively? I think yes. We are able to understand the
impact of our conditioning on the quality of our lives. Dysfunctional
behavior is well recognized today. We can recognize the need for change
and the power of our Original Mind. We can remember how close we
were to our true selves as children. We can recognize the need to nurture
our inner self, our wounded self, and awaken to our original authentic
self. When we do this we have come a long way and have begun our
own "Awakening."

Awareness is the beginning, and cultivation is the work needed to wash
away the dysfunctional thinking. The nurturing of the original self, with
the balance of the energy through the body is part of the cultivation.
The circulation of the Qi through the body is needed to protect and to
evolve into a real human and regain our original real self and obtain
self-realization.

The dualism becomes one within ourselves. We become one in our awareness. Meister Eckhart says:

> I have read many writings both of heathen philosophers and sages…and I have earnestly and with diligence sought the best and highest virtue whereby one may come most closely to God and wherein he may once more become like the original image as he was in God when there was yet no distinction between God and himself before God produced creatures. And having dived into the basis of things to the best of my ability I find that it is no other than absolute detachment from everything that is created…He who would be untouched and pure needs just one thing, 'detachment…'

> If I were perpetually doing God's will, then I would be a virgin in reality, as exempt from idea-handicaps as I was before I was born. (Suzuki p.10-11)

Lao Tzu gives insight into the workings of Tao.

Richard Leirer

Ch 54 Tao Te Ching

When a person embodies Tao -	His heart becomes true
When a Family embodies Tao -	It thrives
When a village embodies Tao -	It is protected
When a country embodies Tao -	It prospers
When the world embodies Tao -	It reveals its perfection

Tao is everywhere
It has become everything
To truly see it, one must see it as
It has revealed itself
In a person, see it as a person
In a family, see it as a family
In a country, see it as a country
In a world, see it as the world.
How have I come to know this?

Tao has shown me.

(Jonathan Star Translation)

Chapter Eight

Ko Wu

考究

The Art of Investigation

Ko Wu means, the art of investigation of life. Socrates is quoted as saying "An unexamined life is not worth living." In reviewing the make-up of our path of cultivation it becomes apparent that a new way of living is being asked of us. We must examine all that we believe to be true and be brave enough to face a world of uncertainty. Liu I-Ming says, "The first priority in cultivating reality is to refine the self and control the mind." (Liu I-Ming p.74)

Having a new life calls for a giving up of the past ideas of who we are and boldly going into a new place of inner awareness. It is this inner awareness that will lead us to a greater understanding of the meaning of life. Tai Chi helps us to become a one-centered person, between heaven and earth, who knows how to be relaxed as a pine tree and uses the hands and mouth in a balanced fashion.

The Wu Chi reminds us that we have unlimited possibilities waiting for us, the possibilities that have not yet arrived in our conscious awareness, waiting to be discovered. Li is the function of the universe and our ability to recognize it inherent in all things. All things inherently have a function or principle. Finding this function or Li, is essential for awakening. Remember, the function of Tai Chi is to become balanced with the yin and yang energies of the universe and align with the Te or virtuous power always present.

Te is the power of the force of the cosmos that is always prompting us into a right and virtuous action. Understanding comes from knowing that the life force or Qi will always be reflecting back that power of Te, if the Qi is in balance within the self.

Releasing the attachments to our conditioned mind is needed in order to let what is natural develop. *Tzu Jan Tao*, the following of what is natural is not available when we engage in "shoulds, musts and have to's." A treatise by Hui-Yuan, "On the explanation of Retribution" says:

> Ignorance is the source of the net of delusion. Greedy
> love is the storehouse for the various mortal ties...
> because ignorance beclouds the understanding,

feeling and thought become clamped to external objects. Because greedy love saturates the nature, the elements cohere to form the body. By their cohering in the body, a boundary comes to be fixed between the I and the not I. By the clamping of feeling, an agent of good and evil arises. If there be a boundary between the I and the not I, the body is then regarded as belonging to the I, and thus cannot be forgotten…a greedy love for life results, so that life can no longer be sundered…The result is that failure and success push after one another, and blessing and calamity follow on each others heels. With the accumulation of evil, divine retribution comes of itself…Thus the retributions of punishment or blessings depend upon what are stimulated by one's own (mental) activities… they result from our own influence.

(Fung Yu – Lan v.2 p.273-274)

The opening of the heart is needed, so the yin and yang energies can become balanced within. When balanced, we can become one with the power of the universe, so we can walk on this earthly plane in a gentle fashion. The methods and tools needed to achieve these goals come with the energy practices and self-awareness that comes from practice.

> There must come a time when one must stop
> repeating the words of others, and stop practicing
> ways of questionable methods, without doing
> some open and honest investigation of the original
> teachings of the Lord Buddha. One must not depend
> on hearsay, or blind belief in what a teacher says,
> simply because he is authority. In the Kalama Sutta,
> the Lord Buddha gives some very wise advice:

> It is unwise to simply believe what one hears
> because it has been said over and over again for a
> long time. It is unwise to follow tradition blindly
> just because it has been practiced in that way for a
> long time. It is unwise to listen to and spread rumors
> and gossip. It is unwise to take anything as being
> the absolute truth just because it agrees with one's
> scriptures (this especially means commentaries and
> sub-commentaries). It is unwise to foolishly make
> assumptions, without investigation. It is unwise to
> abruptly draw a conclusion by what one sees and

hears without further investigation. It is unwise to go by mere outward appearance or to hold too tightly to any view or idea simply because on is comfortable with it. It is unwise to be convinced of anything out of respect and deference to one spiritual teacher (without honest investigation into what is being taught).

We must go beyond opinions, beliefs, and dogmatic thinking. In this way. we can rightly reject anything which when accepted, practiced and perfected, leads to more anger, criticism, conceit, pride, greed, and delusion. These unwholesome states of mind are universally condemned and are certainly not beneficial to ourselves or to others. They are to be avoided whenever possible.

One the other hand, we can rightly accept anything which when practiced and perfected, leads to unconditional love, contentment and gentle wisdom. These things allow us to develop a happy, tranquil, and peaceful mind. Thus, the wise praise all kinds of unconditional love (loving acceptance of the present moment), tranquility, contentment and gentle wisdom and encourages everyone to practice these good qualities as much as possible. (From pages 20 - 21 , The Anapanasati Sutta, Ven. U Vimalaramsi, Published and freely distributed by The Buddhist Association of the United States. May, 2001)

The following are my priorities that help me to investigate my life.

Step one: try to be calm, no matter what is happening be it the good, the bad or the ugly. Calmness is a key to cultivation. There is little chance for success in life if a sense of calmness is not present.

Many of us have never really known what it is like to be calm. From birth, a hectic lifestyle has shown nothing but commotion and often chaos. The typical Western family tries to find calmness watching television or a movie. While this activity breaks our mind away from the struggle of job and family, it does little to create calmness. The types of shows, the noise, the canned laugh tracks, the violence and tragedy as well as the commercials all lead to a tension, not a sense of calmness. So this first step is really the hardest one. It is always a challenge. With 40 years of

Qigong/Tai Chi practice, remaining is still a major task for me.

As long as we are alive, calmness can be a friend to always look for. Modern life can always try to rip away any calmness we do find, often times, within seconds. The tension of a car ride, bad news on the TV or radio, upsetting phone calls, an injustice at work, a snippy family member, are all constant potential robbers of calmness.

The techniques to find calmness are the ones that will work best for you, and discovered by you. Some suggestions include taking a walk in nature, listening to a favorite piece of music, reading a book, poetry, talking with a loved one or friend, meditating, going to church or temple, praying, singing, dancing, creating music, Tai Chi, Qigong, sports, or martial arts. All of these and others can be a source of calmness. The challenge is to find the methods that work for you. Find several. Who you are changes and what is calming will change as you change.

Master Hao Tian You told me:

> Remain calm, even if the mountain above you
> crumbles to dust; remain calm even if the earth below
> you opens and tries to swallow you, remain calm. Not

wanting the mountain to crumble and not wanting the earth to open might not be enough to stop it from happening anyway. What can be controlled are our own selves. Remain calm.

The second goal in cultivation is to not take things personally. This concept is well outlined in Chapter 2. of *"The Four Agreements"* by Don Miguel Ruiz.

Basically the principle is this: no matter what another says or does, do not take it personally. That other is creating their perception of you at that moment. It may or may not be accurate. You may not accurately perceive the true meaning of what another is trying to say either. However, "When you take things personally, then you feel offended, and your reaction is to defend your beliefs and create conflicts." (Ruiz p.50)

Communicating anything, particularly from and to a loved one, is a great challenge. The opportunity for miscommunication is great. Deborah Tannen (*I Only Say This Because I Love You* and *You Just Don't Understand*) has done a great deal of work giving examples of how miscommunication is the rule of the day.

The metamessages that are sent in many conversations in the course of a day change from what was said, to what was meant to be said, and finally to how it was received.

> A metamessage is meaning that is not said – at least not in so many words – but that we glean from every aspect of context: the way something is said, who is saying it, or the fact that it is said at all. (Tannen p.7)

Wow, imagine how many metamessages we are all bombarded with, on a regular basis? Remember the frustration that comes from not being heard because someone received a metamessage (sent or not). Observe the anger that can come from hearing others' metamessages (sent or not).

Keeping in mind the first goal is to remaining calm, it is easier to understand why this is so important and so difficult at the same time. The second goal of not taking things personally reminds us all, that what we think is going on might not be accurate.

Sometimes metamessages can lead to a "Mutually Aggravating Spiral, which each person's response drives the other to more extreme forms of the opposing behavior." (Tannen p.103.)

Tannen uses a term "complementary schismogenesis," coined by Gregory Bateson, an anthropologist, to describe this mutually aggravating spiral. "Suppose one person tends to speak slightly more loudly than another. The softer speaker may speak even more softly to encourage the other to follow suit, while the louder speaker speaks even more loudly to encourage the whisperer to speak up. Each time one adjusts the volume to set a good example, the other intensifies the opposing behavior, until one is whispering and the other is shouting, both exaggerating their styles." (Tannen p.103)

Sometimes this "Mutually Aggravating Spiral" leads to a wanting from another a behavior as noted above. It could also be a wanting of an apology and the not getting it or many other types of controlling behavior. Remembering how we perceive the universe and how others do is part of conditioning. Our conditioned minds, expecting certain behaviors, bump into others conditioned thinking. Remembering not to take things personally helps in communicating by dissuading " Mutually Aggravating Spiral" situations from unfolding.

Defaulting to a thought "This is just my conditioned thinking and that is just theirs," goes a long way in keeping calm. Learning and practicing to carefully choose words and phrases that accurately reflect what you mean goes a long way. Paraphrasing back what you heard is also a helpful to keep confusion to a minimum.

Even if communication finally does take place, and you clearly hear what the other is saying, who is to say who's message is more important. What do you do with the message that is in conflict with your own? Above all, do not take it personally. Remain removed from a personal connection that the opinion is a judgment about yourself. It is just an idea or thought from another person. Your original mind knows who and what you are. Others might not.

Learn to listen to what comes up from within you as you attempt to communicate with others. Great lessons can be found in this type of exchange.

The third goal is to become aware of self-esteem issues. Virginia Satir, family therapist and author of *The New Peoplemaking* says,

No matter what kind of problem first led a family

into my office ... I soon found that the prescription was the same. To relieve their family pain, some way had to be found to challenge these four key factors. In all troubled families I noticed that:

1) Self – worth was low.

2.) Communication was indirect, vague and not really honest.

3.) Rules were rigid, inhuman, nonnegotiable, and everlasting.

4.) The families' link to society was fearful, placating, and blaming.   (Satir p.04)

These stumbling blocks to finding the true self are ingrained in our consciousness. If my self worth is low, of course I am going to take things personally.

If communication is vague, indirect and not really honest, how do I know how to connect with another or how another would see who I really am? I will have to guess. Most of the time I will guess incorrectly, and I might think whatever is wrong must be my fault. Since everything is my fault and I am to blame I must be an unworthy person who has broken the rules. I wasn't correct. I misbehaved. I did something wrong. Not only do I know it, so does everybody else. Since I must have broken some rule, I deserve to be punished. After all, you make your bed, you lie in it. These are the attitudes of conditioning and must be overcome so we can become truly our best.

Marshal Rosenberg calls this type of thinking a Jackal. We can Jackal ourselves inwardly, or Jackal others outwardly. The language goes like this:

> At an early age, most of us were taught to speak and think Jackal. This is a moralistic classification idiom that labels people; it has a splendid vocabulary for analyzing and criticizing. Jackal is good for telling people what's wrong with them: 'Obviously, you're emotionally disturbed (rude, lazy, selfish).' The jackal moves close to the ground. It is so preoccupied with getting its immediate needs met that it cannot see into the future. Similarly Jackal-thinking individuals believe that in quickly classifying or analyzing people, they understand them. Unhappy about what's going on, a Jackal will label the people

involved, saying, 'He's an idiot' or 'She's bad' or 'They're culturally deprived.'   (Rosenberg p.01)

Rosenburg also discovered a language of the heart. This would be language coming from the original self, not the conditioned self. He describes it like this:

> I also came upon a language of the heart, a form of interactingthatpromotesthewell-beingofourselvesand other people. I call this means of communicating Giraffe. The Giraffe has the largest heart of any land animal, is tall enough to look into the future, and lives its life with gentility and strength. Likewise, Giraffe bids us to speak from the heart, to talk about what is going on for us – without judging others. In this idiom, you give people an opportunity to say yes, although you respect no for an answer. Giraffe is a language of requests; Jackal is a language of demands. (ibid)

Learning the language of non violent communication as outlined above by Rosenberg gives another tool in awareness and self cultivation. As awareness of language increases, awareness of the goodness of the self also increases.

Step four is all about forgiveness. Forgiveness of the self is needed in order to be skilled at forgiving others. The idea that I will do something wrong, or its always my fault can hinder cultivation. How can I forgive myself if I have done so many horrible things in the past? Remind yourself you did the best you could with what you knew. Now you know better and can eflect on errors, make corrections and offer forgiveness to yourself and others. With the skill of forgiveness, it becomes easier to connect with others. Knowing others did the best they knew how to do helps jump-start the forgiveness mechanism inside. Being gentle with yourself leads to being gentle with others.

The fifth step is developing the habit of daily review of how your life has been. This review is as follows:

1) Recognition of mistakes, Review what happened during the day that you feel responsible for or feel uncomfortable about. Trust that your original mind will remind you, of what actions undertaken in the course of a day that do not sit well in your mind. This review is best done at night as we prepare for sleep. Do not judge or explain or defend what arises in your mind. Let the mind be free to examine

the day without recrimination of any kind.

2) Quiet the heart. This technique uses a willingness to allow heart/mind to be quiet and still. Because the heart is not still, mind is active. Still and quiet the heart, and the mind will follow. Ask yourself, "What is it that upsets my heart today?" After a few minutes of listening, ask your heart to become calm. Simply request it to do so. It will follow and comply with your request. Usually the heart will revert back to the recognition of the mistakes made during the day and a wish to correct them. Allow this to happen, do not censure.

3) Develop a gentle understanding towards yourself and others. As your heart finds what worries it has, listen with a gentle understanding. Most of us have an internal critic that is anything but gentle. That internal critic will beat up and put down and criticize in the harshest and cruelest way. To counter this attack, a gentle inner nurturer is needed.

One way to find this inner nurturer is to think of yourself as a very old and wise person. See yourself as someone who has lived a full life and has the wisdom to see events from a lifetime perspective. That person will be gentle, loving and caring towards you if you allow it. Many of us may shudder at this thought. However, after awhile, this inner wise sage will become a friend and companion to console you in all that life brings you. This nurturer will help you develop gentleness towards yourself, particularly your faults and weaknesses. As you become gentle with yourself you will become gentle with others. Even if you still think and feel that they are wrong, dumb, stupid or even mean. The heart and wise nurturer knows this is Jackal talk and it will naturally shift to Giraffe speak on its own.

4) Develop the ability to forgive yourself and others. Make this a daily habit.

5) Make restitution towards yourself and others. When doing the daily review, it is sometimes apparent that we have hurt someone or injured someone or falsely accused someone or harmed our self or others. After quieting our heart, forgiving, and understanding, there is still the need for corrective action for our behavior. Use this time to develop a plan to make restitution for actions performed. Your wise nurturer can be called upon to develop the how to of getting it done. This is an essential role in our cultivation. Making amends and restitution is a big step in taking responsibility for our actions. With responsibility will come natural and logical consequences we will easily recognize and use to change future

behavior.

6) Resolve and state an affirmation to manifest the original nature within the self. Daily, affirm the original self that lies within and give permission for it to make itself an active part of your life. Remember, each of us is a part of the Wu Chi, a Child of God and the Universe.

Remembering Max Ehrmann's poem, *Desiderata*:

>Go placidly amidst the noise and haste, and remember what peace there may be in silence. As far as possible without surrender be on good terms with all persons. Speak your truth quietly and clearly; and listen to others, even the dull and the ignorant; they too have their story.
>
>Avoid loud and aggressive persons, they are vexatious to the spirit. If you compare yourself with others, you may become vain or bitter; for always there will be greater and lesser persons than yourself.
>
>Enjoy your achievements as well as your plans. Keep

interested in your own career, however humble; it is a real possession in the changing fortunes of time.

Exercise caution in your business affairs; for the world is full of trickery. But let this not blind you to what virtue there is; many persons strive for high ideals; and everywhere life is full of heroism.

Be yourself. Especially, do not feign affection. Neither be cynical about love; for in the face of all aridity and disenchantment it is as perennial as the grass.

Take kindly the counsel of the years, gracefully surrendering the things of youth. Nurture strength of spirit to shield you in sudden misfortune. But do not distress yourself with dark imaginings. Many fears are born of fatigue and loneliness.

Beyond a wholesome discipline, be gentle with yourself. *You are a child of the universe, no less than the trees and the stars; you have a right to be here.*

And whether or not it is clear to you, no doubt the

universe is unfolding as it should. Therefore be at peace with God, whatever you conceive Him to be, and whatever your labours and aspirations, in the noisy confusion of life keep peace with your soul. With all its shams, drudgery, and broken dreams, it is still a beautiful world. Be cheerful. Strive to be happy

The Chinese Sages say. "In all the world there is nothing greater than the tip of an autumn hair; Mount T'ai is small". If all things conform to their inner nature and accept their limitations then what is large does not single out its largeness nor does what is small single out its smallness. Adequacy in one's one nature is what is great. Then divine nature can be claimed. Qigong/Tai Chi training provides the discipline, energy, knowledge and understanding of the natural workings of the universe to create a self realized person.

Chapter Nine

Qigong & Tai Chi Forms to Practice
氣功和太極拳的形式實踐

A Brief History of Qigong and Tai Chi

Qigong has a long history in China going back to Emperor Yao [2356-2255 B.C.E.] There are also Bronze era objects with Qigong inscriptions dating from the Zhou Dynasty of the 11th century B.C.-771 B.C.E. In ancient times Qigong went by different names such as *XinQi* (promoting and conducting Qi), *FuQi* (taking Qi), *Tuna* (Inhale/Exhale), *Daoyin* (Inducing and conducting Qi), *AnQiao* (Massage), *Shushu* (Breath Counting), *Jingzuo* or *Jing Gong* (Sitting Still), and *Wogong* (Lying Down Exercises). (See *Bi Yong Sheng* et al.p. 2)

One of the key components of these exercises is an underlying concept of man in his relationship to the natural world. This is summed up by an old saying, "man is related with heaven and earth, and corresponds with the sun and the moon," taken from Chapter 79 of the *Miraculous Pivot*, an ancient health text. (Sun Guangren et.al p.26) The natural world teaches us about balance and how to stay healthy through exercise. Hua Tuo, a physician and healer, who created the five-animal frolics over 2,000 years ago, developed those exercises by watching animals like a tiger, bear, deer, monkey and birds.

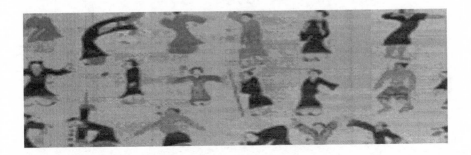

The first use of the word Tai Chi goes back to its use in the *I Ching* from 3rd to the 2nd millennium B.C. The concept of the balance of yin and yang is pivotal in understanding Chinese Philosophy and the Tai Chi concept. As a concept Tai Chi has this ancient root. The actual physical practice of Tai Chi, as opposed to Qigong practices mentioned above begins about the 12 th century A.D.

The beginnings of Tai Chi as we know it today is a controversial issue. Some say Tai Chi was created by the Chen family in the 1600's. I believe it was created by Taoist (Daoist) internal arts and Master Zhang, San-Feng in the 1200's. We know that Zhang, San Feng was born in 1242 AD., and might have lived until the 1400's. Legends say he was a healer and a sage as well as the founder of the internal school of Tai Chi practiced at Wudang Shan.

Some say he is a myth and never really existed, because he is said to have lived so long. Those that do not believe he founded Tai Chi fail to realize that there are records of his birth. There is also evidence for his contributions to the internal schools as early as 1669. In an Epitaph for Wang, Zhang-Nan (1669) a famous Martial Artist which said:

> Shaolin School 少林 was worldly prominent by its pugilism...there was something called the Internal School... began with Zhang, San-Feng 張三峰 of Song dynasty, and San-Feng was an alchemist of Wudang Mountains.

This indicates Zhang, San-Feng had already been recognized for his contributions in the Martial Arts world at this time in history.

Zhang, San-Feng, like the early Qigong styles mentioned above also developed his exercise of Tai Chi by observing the natural world. Seeing the interplay of a snake and a crane, he developed the movements of Tai Chi following the yin and yang of their movements. When the crane would strike with its beak, the snake would withdraw and coil. Seeing the

143

crane over stretched with its beak out in attack, the snake unfurled and shot straight toward the crane. The crane, sensing the attack, withdraws and opens its wings. Back and forth the battle ensued until both tired and went their separate ways, only to return at a later time. The Tai Chi movements of Snake Creeps Down and White Crane Flash Wings comes directly from this observation. The rest of the Tai Chi movements reflect the yin, inward, coiled motion or the straight, outward and yang expanding motions.

Dr. Yang, Jwing-Ming says,

> Taijiquan (Tai Chi Chuan) is an internal style of martial arts that was created in the Daoist monastery of the Wudang mountain, Hubei Province. Taijiquan's creation was based on the philosophies of Taiji and Yin-Yang. It is believed that from understanding the theory of Taiji and Yin-Yang, we will be able to trace back the origin of our lives. Also, through this understanding, we will be able to train our bodies correctly, to maintain our health and the strength of our physical and energetic bodies, and gain longevity. Since Daoists are monks, the final goal of their spiritual

cultivation is to reunite with the natural spirit, the state of Wuji. In order to reach this goal, they must cultivate their human nature and nourish it (discipline their temperament).

For a well written argument about the authenticity of Zhang, San Feng as the founder of Tai Chi see http://ymaa.com/articles/origin-of-taijiquan and a great article written by David Silver.

Richard Leirer

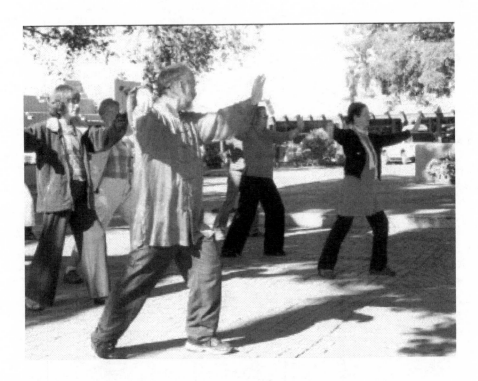

Tai Chi Practice in Taos Plaza, New Mexico

Qigong and Tai Chi Forms

QIGONG WARM-UP EXERCISE
MOVEMENTS FOR HEALTH

**Stand with feet shoulder width apart, knees slightly bent.
Repeat each exercise eight times, unless otherwise noted.**

Opening Movement

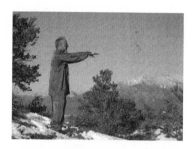

- Slowly raise hands to shoulder level, moving from shoulder to fingertips - fingertips extending
- Inhale as your arms rise – exhale as the arms fall
- Open the joints as the arms rise – from the toes up through ankle – knee- hips – spine – out shoulder – elbow – wrists – to fingers
- When breathing in, open and feel Chi, like air pass, thru the joints
- When breathing out and closing, feel Chi pack into the joints as you pull your arms back, dropping the elbow and pushing the hands downward till the thumbs touch the thigh.
- Repeat eight times then continue with the hands rising in a V pattern to open the chest and back wing bone area for another eight times.

147

Richard Leirer

LIKE A BIRD (Simple stretch)

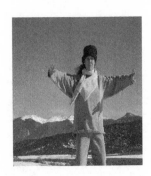

- Cross arms in front of the body.
- Gently swing arms out from the shoulders.
- Bend elbows slightly & push palms out to sides
    (Breathe in as you cross your arms in front, breathe out
    as they extend to sides.)

ELBOW TO THE SKY

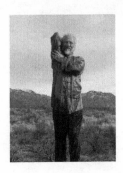

- Raise right arm curling *first* the wrist, *then* the elbow.
- Place curved wrist on the shoulder pointing the elbow to the
  sky.
- Gently lower arm, uncurling first the elbow, then the wrist.
    (Breathe in as the arm is raised, breathe out as it is lowered.)
- Repeat with left arm.

SHRUG THE SHOULDERS

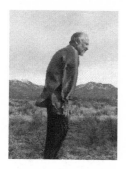

- Bring the shoulders up towards the ears.
- Gently roll the shoulders forward, rotating the arms inward.
- As you lean slightly forward, slide the hands, palms facing out, down the front of the thighs to just above the knees.
- As you straighten up, the hands slide back up the thighs.
- Gently roll the shoulders back and down.
(Breathe in as you bring the shoulders to the ears, breathe out as you lean forward. Breathe in as you straighten up, breathe out as you roll the shoulders back & down.)

GIVE YOURSELF A HUG

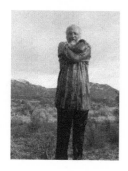

- Breathing in, swing your arms out to the sides at shoulder level.
- Breathe out swinging your arms across the body to give yourself a hug.

- Give yourself verbal affirmations like:
I have a great memory
I have a great immune system
I am loved and I am lovable

LIKE A BUTTERFLY

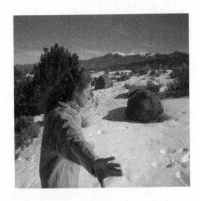

- Extend both arms out in front, a slight bend in the elbow.
- Swing arms back, keeping the elbows bent so the hands dangle.
- Tuck hands, wrists bending, under the armpits and move them forward with palms facing up.
(Breathe in as arms swing back, breathe out as hands move forward.)
- **Reverse -** from palms up position, draw the hands in to the armpits, then swing them out to the sides, elbows slightly bent, hands dangling, until the edges of hands meet in front.
- Turn palms up and repeat.

THE WAVE

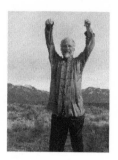

- Swing both arms up in front, wrists relaxed, fingers pointing down.
- Let both arms glide down, palms facing outward, and fingers pointing up for as long as possible.
  (Breathe in as arms swing up, breathe out as they glide down)

UNLOCKING THE FROZEN GATE

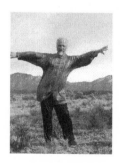

- Gently and slowly rotate the hips forward, then to the right, to the back, to the left, then forward, making a complete circle.
- Knees should move as little as possible. Make 6 circles.
- **Reverse** direction. Make 6 circles. (Breathe normally)

Classic Eight Best Movements for Health
Plus More

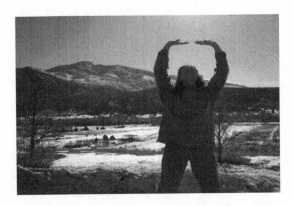

TWO HANDS HOLD THE SKY

1. Feet shoulder width apart. Knees relaxed, slightly bent.
2. Bring hands together in front, palms facing abdomen. Move hands forward, turning palms upward.
3. Move hands back toward abdomen, palms up, then make an outward circle with hands dangling from the wrists.
4. When hands meet at forehead, interlace fingers and turn palms upward.
5. Shift weight to balls of feet and reach for the sky, keeping a slight bend in the elbow.
6. Release fingers and move hands in a downward circle, palms facing out, until they meet at the starting point in front of the abdomen.
7. Lower heels as you move hands downwards.

REPEAT EIGHT TIMES

Benefits
This exercise regulates internal organs: the heart and lungs in the upper

torso, the kidneys and intestines in the lower abdomen. It relieves fatigue, invigorates the muscles and bones of the back and waist, and helps correct poor posture.

BEND THE BOW AND SHOOT THE ARROW

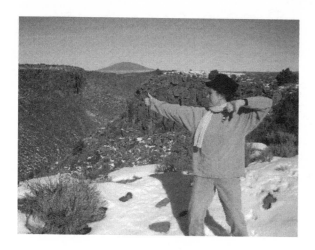

1. Feet shoulder width apart. Knees relaxed, slightly bent.
2. Raise right hand to touch left shoulder.(Reach for bow.)
3. Circle right hand over the head - circle left hand - hands meet in center. (Arrow meets the bow.)
4. Move right hand to the right, palm facing front. Pull left elbow back, keeping the elbow bent, palm facing front. (Shooting the arrow.) Keep eyes on right hand.
5. Lower right hand to the side.
6. Raise left hand to touch right shoulder.
7. Circle left hand - circle right hand - hands meet in center.
8. Move left hand to the left, palm facing front. Push right elbow back, keeping elbow bent, palm facing the front. (Shooting the arrow.)
   Keep eyes on left hand.

REPEAT EIGHT TIMES

Benefits
This exercise expands the chest, improving the circulation of blood and oxygen, and improves the flow of Chi.

WAVING HEAD AND TAIL

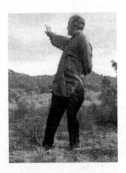

1.   Feet shoulder width apart, knees relaxed and slightly bent.
2.   Fingertips of left hand come together to form a tail.
3.   Turn body and arms to the left, bending the knees. Move left hand to the lower back and leave there as a tail.
4.   Move right hand to the right as far as you can turn. Palm hand faces away from you and at eye level, elbow is bent. Watch back of hand.
5.   Turn palm to face you. Move right hand to the left as far as you can turn, elbow is bent. Watch palm of hand.
6.   Drop both arms & turn torso to right, bending the knees. Right hand becomes a bird's tail by wrapping fingers around the thumb. Move right hand to the lower back and leave it there as a tail.
7.   Move left hand to the left as far as you can turn. Palm of hand faces away from you and at eye level, elbow is bent. Watch back of left hand.

8.   Turn palm to face you. Move left hand to right as far as you can turn, elbow bent. Watch palm of hand. Drop arms, turn back.

REPEAT EIGHT TIMES

Benefits

This exercise is potent. It has a powerful effect on the nervous system and the circulation of blood and Chi. It helps relieve heartburn, stimulates the power of the kidneys, strengthens the eyeballs and the muscles of the neck and shoulders. It is excellent for alleviating high blood pressure.

TENSE AND PUNCH

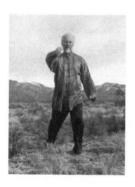

1.   Move left foot forward (heel down, roll onto toes).
2.   Right foot is kept flat. Heel stays on ground. Circle wave in with left hand.
3.   Punch with right hand (left knee is bent forward). Rock back. Pull left hand back like retreat repulse monkey.
4.   Move left foot back to the instep, then to the side.
5.   Move right foot to the instep, then forward (heel down, roll onto toes).
6.   Left foot is kept flat. Heel stays on ground. Wave in with right hand.

7. Punch with left hand (right knee is bent forward). Rock back.
8. Move right foot back to the instep, then to the side.

REPEAT EIGHT TIMES

Benefits

This exercise develops the flow of Chi from your feet through your entire body. This is *NOT* a punching exercise – it is designed to strengthen the flow of internal power. It must be done slowly and calmly.

TWO HANDS HOLD THE FEET

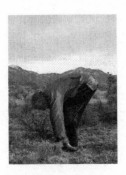

1. Feet shoulder width apart. Knees relaxed, slightly bent.
2. Round the back, Chin to the chest.
3. Slide hands down outside of body as you bend forward.
4. Move hands around the toes, then up inside of legs.
5. Bend knees, push hips forward, lift up, bend backwards, raising arms over head and out to sides, keeping elbows bent.

REPEAT EIGHT TIMES

Benefits

This exercise is good for muscles of the lower back and legs and for stretching the spine. It benefits the stomach and lower abdomen, strengthens the kidneys and bladder.

LOOK AT OPPOSITE HEEL

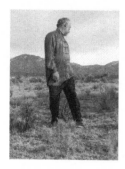

1.   Feet shoulder width apart. Knees relaxed, slightly bent.
2.   Arms hang loosely at the sides.
3.   While bending the knees, turn body slowly to the left and look at right heel.
4.   Turn body slowly to the right, bending the knees, and look at left heel.
5.   Do not lean.

REPEAT EIGHT TIMES

Benefits
This exercise has a powerful relaxing effect. It strengthens the flow of Chi, and Master Huang Tseng Yu says it eases tiredness and hurt.

RAISING SINGLE HAND

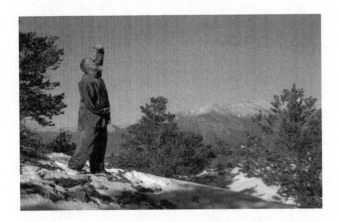

1. Feet shoulder width apart, knees relaxed, slightly bent.
2. Using a scooping motion, raise right hand to mouth (as if taking a drink).
3. Turn palm of right hand toward the sky as you raise the right hand directly over the head. (The heel of the right hand should be slightly higher than the fingers.)
4. Make 1/2 circle out to the right side with right arm, elbow slightly bent. The eyes follow the movement of the hand.
5. Using a scooping motion, raise left hand to mouth (as if taking a drink).
6. Turn palm of left hand toward the sky as you raise the left hand directly over the head. (The heel of the left hand will be slightly higher than the fingers.)
7. Make 1/2 circle with the left hand. The eyes follow the movement of the hand.

REPEAT EIGHT TIMES

Benefits

The movements in this exercise increase the flow of Chi along both sides of the body and benefit the liver, gall, spleen and stomach.

LIKE A TURTLE

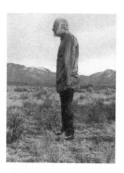

1.   Feet shoulder width apart, knees relaxed, slightly bent.
2.   Push your Chin forward.
3.   Gently and slowly move the Chin in a horizontal circle.
4.   Reverse direction.
      (Begin with 4 circles in each direction, gradually building up to 8.)

Benefits
This exercise loosens the neck, exercising the cervical vertebra. It promotes drainage of lymph in the head and neck.

LIKE A SWAN

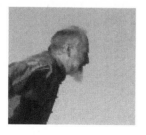

1.   Feet shoulder width apart. Knees relaxed, slightly bent.

159

2.   Push the Chin forward.
3.   Move the Chin down, then back toward the chest, then up, then forward. (Making a vertical circle, like a Ferris wheel.)
4.   Reverse direction.
         (Begin with 4 circles in each direction, gradually building to 8.)

Benefits

This exercise also loosens the neck, exercising the cervical vertebrae. Relieves headache.

YIJINJING

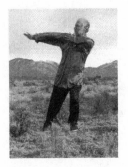

Part A.
1.   Raise arms from the sides to shoulder level, palms down.
2.   Bend right elbow, extend the left arm.
3.   Turn head to watch extending arm.
4.   Turning head back to right, bend left elbow and extend right arm.
5.   Repeat eight times, then turn palms up and repeat another eight times.

(You can begin with four each palms up, palms down and gradually work up to eight or more repetitions.)

Benefits
Loosens and unfreezes the shoulder, the rotator cuff and under the arm.
Also exercises the wrist and upper arm.

LIMBERING THE WINGS

1. Let arms hang loosely at the sides.
2. Place left hand on the chest under the collar bone. Fold the right shoulder forward allowing the arm to follow naturally. The palm will turn outward as the arm rotates.
3. Slowly unfold the shoulder as far back as it will go and relax it.
   Repeat with left shoulder.

REPEAT EIGHT OR MORE TIMES

Benefits
Exercises the shoulders and the scapulae. Helps prevent upper respiratory infections, treats the lungs, opens the pulmonary pathways.

YIJINJING
Part B.

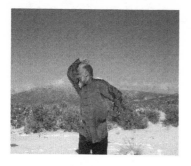

1. Circle the right hand, palm up, toward the body and under the arm.

2. While shifting the weight to the left leg, extend the right hand out from under the arm as far as it will go without locking the elbow, still palm up.

3. Straighten up, turn the right palm over (up), bend the elbow and repeat
Repeat 3 or 4 times with each arm. Then continue with both arms.

4. Both arms at one time: While circling the right hand inward and shifting your weight to the left leg, bring the left hand up to guard the right side of the face, palm facing to the right. Extend right arm to the right as in #2 above.

5. Straighten up and repeat on left side, shifting the weight to the right leg.

WORK UP TO 8
REPETITIONS

Part C

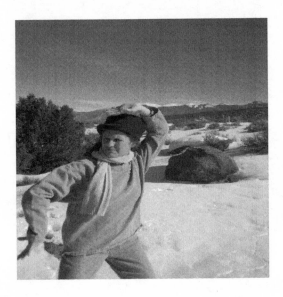

1.   With palm of one hand facing the sky, circle the hand inward (toward the body) and under the arm and then move the arm upwards.

2.   Circle the hand (palm still facing the sky) above the head, then lower the hand back down and circle under the arm again.

Start out with three or four repetitions and gradually work up to eight.

Remember to reverse direction and repeat.

3.   Then do the same exercise with the other arm.

4.   Then move arms at the same time.

WORK UP TO 8
REPETITIONS

Benefits

Opens the shoulder, rotator cuff and increases blood circulation to the head, heart and arms.

WEEPING WILLOW QUIVERS IN THE COOL BREEZE

1.   Feet shoulder width apart. Knees relaxed, slightly bent.

2.   Start a gentle vibration of the body, working up from the ankles, to the knees, hips, spine.

3.   Concentrate the vibration into each disc and vertebra of the spine starting a the tailbone, moving upwards, like climbing the rungs of a ladder, until you reach the base of the skull.

4.   Then move up the back of the head to one side of the brain. Gently vibrate that side of the brain, then the eye, ear, nose and throat on that side of that head. Then switch to the other side and repeat.

5.   Allow the vibration to move out of the sides and back of the neck to the shoulder muscles, to the rotators, then

down to the elbows, wrists and fingers.

6.   Vibrate the abdominal cavity and then the chest cavity.

7.   Allow your mind to move the vibration into the liver (the energy of the east, the wood element, shaking out anger and shaking in kindness), the heart,(the energy of the south and the element of Fire, shaking out sorrow and cruelty-shaking in joy and happiness), the spleen and pancreas,(the energy of the center, the element of earth, shaking out worry and anxiety-shaking in compassion), lungs,(the energy of the west, the element of metal, shaking out sadness and grief and shaking in courage), kidneys and adrenals(the energy of the north, the element of water, shaking out fear and shaking in gentleness).

8.   Concentrate the gentle vibration into the abdominal space, relaxing the entire abdominal cavity. Include the stomach, intestines, the ovaries or testes and prostate.

9.   Gently vibrate the whole body. Feel the inner organs vibrate.
Roll your weight onto the balls of the feet. Move your body up and down.
(If legs get tired, put heels down on the floor, but keep moving up and down)

10.   As you increase your stamina, advance to doing small jumps.

Gradually work up to doing 64 small jumps.

Benefits

Refreshes and regenerates all the internal organs by enabling them to massage each other. It is also excellent for the spine and nervous system and your sense of balance. It tends to remove all sickness.

24 FORM TAI CHI CHUAN

Helpful Reminders for ease of practice and Maximum Results

1) You must stand with the head as if suspended from the sky by a string at the top of the head. The tongue must touch the roof of the mouth, connecting the Ren and Tu Mai acupuncture channels.

2) The Tailbone must point down. Do not let the tailbone sway back. Chi energy will leak out if this happens.

3) The knees must have a slight bend in them. As your strength increases, your bent knee position can also increase.

4) The joints must remain loose and open.

5) Every movement must be connected.

6) Every movement must be continuous. Keep moving, do not pause, hesitate, or stop until you reach the conclusion.

7) Breathe in and out through the nose. At the beginning of learning Tai Chi do not worry about how to breathe. Just let the breathing be natural. After 3-5 years of practicing Tai Chi working with breathe can begin. Generally when a movement is towards the body breath in, movement away from the body breath out.

After an even longer time of practice (8-10 yrs) reverse abdominal breathing can be applied. Do not try to go too slowly. This short form will take about 3-5 minutes to perform. If you take longer than 5 min, it is probably too slow.

8) All forward steps move in and then out, like the shape of a sideways V. However, the front foot must point straight.

9) Square shoulders and hips to the direction you are traveling.

10) All forward steps lead with the heel first, all backwards steps with the toe first, all sideways steps with the toe first.

11) There are only four types of steps in this form: forward, backward, sideways and a half forward step. In the half step, drag the instep of the back foot toward the heel of the front foot and do a step ball change. Shift the weight to the ball of the back dragged foot and allow the front foot to raise like a cat, heel up.

12) Double weighedness must be avoided. This means weight is shifting from one foot to another continuously, and not held balanced between the two. It also means that the front foot must be to the left or right of the heel of the back foot. Imagine drawing a line forward from the heel of your back foot. Your forward foot must be on the opposite side of your back foot. If your right foot is back, the left foot will be forward and to the left of your right heel and that extended imaginary line. If the left foot is back, the right foot must be to the right of the back left heel. To get the correct stepping posture, look in the direction you will be stepping. If the left foot is going to step, extend your left arm, aligned with your back heel and pointing to the direction you will be stepping.

Then make sure the left foot steps to the left of your extended arm. Readjust the back foot to the 45-degree angle.

13) The back heel must stay connected to the ground. Do not let it leave the ground until you are moving forward to the next movement.

14) The leading hand must go to the strike zone within the frame of the body. Generally the strike zone is the physical width of the body, extending from the bridge of the nose down to the bottom of the breastbone. All leading hands must stay within this strike zone. Do not let them go outside the frame of the body.

15) All movements generate at the waist, generally moving into the feet and then into the hands. Remember, the tail does not wag the dog. This means the hands do not lead a movement.

16). The mind leads the Chi through the nine holed pearl. The mind thinks the Chi moves through the ankle, knee, hip, tailbone (*wei lu*), small of back (*ming men*), wing bone (*jiaji*), shoulder, elbow, wrist into palm.

Embrace Tiger, Return to Mountain

..The Essence Of Tai Chi

If I continually reach out to others for love,
I am tipping forward, off-center and unstable,
leaning on whomever I contact
and likely to fall flat and hard if the other leaves.

If I continually withdraw in fear,
I am tipping backward, tense and rigid
and the slightest surprise will push me over.

If I feel uncertain in myself
and unstable in my base,
then all my contacts with others
will be wobbly and lack conviction.

If I can become centered and balanced
in my own experience,
then I carry this moving center with me.

If I am balanced now… Then I can move in any
direction I wish with no danger of falling, and my
contact with you is solid and real, coming to

you…from the root of my living.

Chungliang Al Huang

24 FORM TAI CHI CHUAN

Form 1   **Beginning (Commencing) Form**

• Begin with heels together, toes at a 45 degree angle (like a Penguin). Move left foot to your left. At this point, feet need to be shoulder width apart, knees slightly bent.

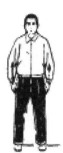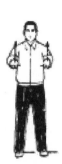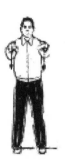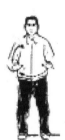

• Allow arms to slowly rise forward to about waist level, then let them gently sink until thumbs touch the thighs. (Hands to the back)

• Move weight to balls of feet and allow arms to drift upward, extending fingers and turning palms toward the abdomen (dantian area). Find your ball or silky bubble, and shift weight back to whole foot. Sink down.

• Turn the ball over (right hand on top) while turning on the left toe and step out with the left foot.

Form   2   Part the Horse's Mane   (3 times)

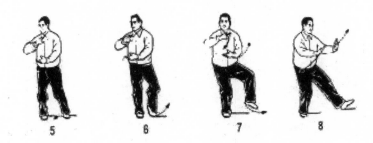

• As left foot steps out, left hand rises, palm up; right hand descends to hip level, palm down.

• Rock back. Hold the ball over the left hip, step forward with right foot, right hand rises, palm up; left hand descends to hip level, palm down.

• Rock back. Hold ball over right hip, step forward left foot; left hand rises, palm up; right hand descends to hip level, palm down.

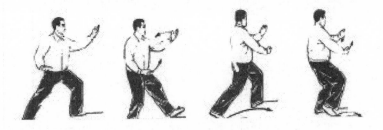

Part the Wild Horses Mane three times

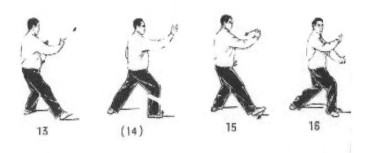

13   (14)   15   16

Form 3   White Crane Flashes Its Wings

• As right foot drags forward, left hand sinks down next
to left hip, palm facing down, while right hand moves up to about eye
level, and palm flashes forward. Turn the waist to the right allowing the
arms to turn with the waist, but not changing the arm position.

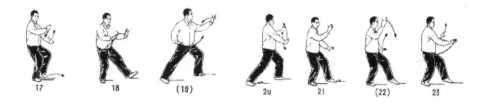

17   18   (19)   20   21   (22)   23

• Turn palms over. While turning waist to the left, left
hand rises and right hand descends to cross in front of the
body at waist level, palm down.
• Turn palms over. While turning waist back to the right,
right hand rises and left hand crosses in front of the body,
palm down.

Form 4 Brush Knee (3 times) (Start on left side)

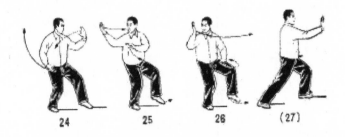

- Step out left foot and brush left knee with left palm, right palm pushes forward.

- Rock back. Hold the ball over the left hip; step out with right foot and brush right knee with right palm as left hand pushes forward. Rock back. Hold the ball over the right hip.

- Step out with left foot and brush left knee, right palm pushes.

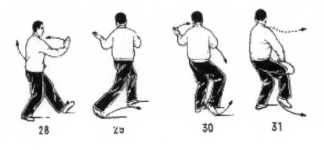

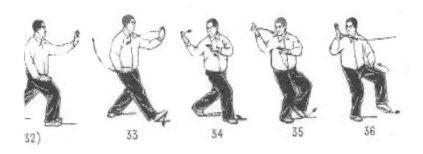

(Drag right foot 1/2 step & shift weight to back foot after third brush to start next movement.

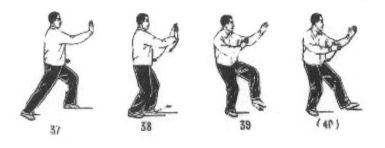

Form   5   Hands Come Up In 7 Stars/Strum the Lute

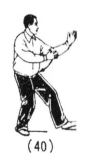

(40)

Strum the lute or play the guitar or Pi Pa. The relaxed left hand rises to hold the lute. Right hand strums the strings downward.

(Right hand, palm facing up, pulls back at the waist and extends behind you to start next form. When downward hand passes hip, palm turns upward to start Retreat Repulse Monkey, (also known as Step Back and Whirl Arms on Both Sides (4 times).

Form 6   Step Back and Whirl Arms on Both Sides (4 times)
Retreat Repulse Monkey

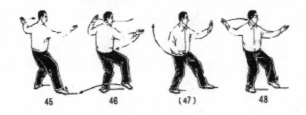

When right hand passes the right hip, turn the waist to the right so as to look at the back hand. Left hand has to remain out in front.

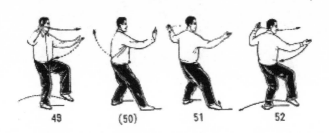

- Turn palms up, bend elbows

- Right hand pushes past the right ear.

- Step back left foot as left hands pulls back at the waist, extending behind you.

- Turn waist as you watch left hand float gently up behind you, keeping the wrist relaxed.

- Repeat right side. Repeat left side. Repeat right side.

- Turn body 1/4 turn to the right, drawing the left foot into the right instep. Hold ball over right hip

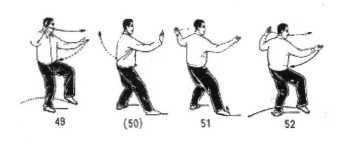

49 (50) 51 52

(Step on the diagonal with the left foot to start the next movement)

Form 7 Grasp Bird's Tail - Left Side

- As you step out, left arm rises, palm facing you.

Right hand rises, palm up, to meet left hand. (Palms face each other, but do not touch.)

175

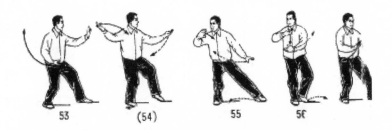

53 (54) 55 56

• Rock back and pull both hands back in a downward arc on right side.

• Turn right hand so fingers point to the sky (hands would then make a plus (+) sign), then push both hands forward, palms still facing each other but not touching.

• Hands separate to make a reverse circle above the shoulders, one in front of each shoulder, moving downward towards the waist.

•Push both hands forward.

(Rock back and turn 180°)

Form   8   Grasp Bird's Tail - Right Side

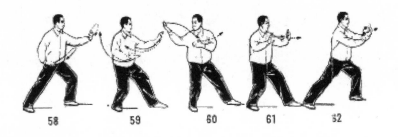

58   59   60   61   62

• As right foot steps out, right hand rises, palm facing you.

• Left arm rises, palm up, to meet right hand. (Palms face each other, but does not touch have to touch.)

•Repeat as in Form 7, above.

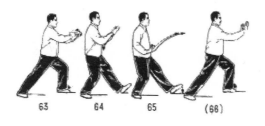

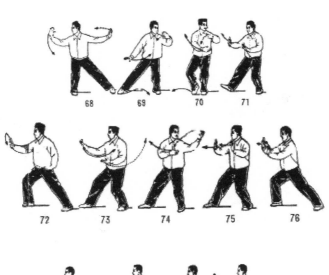

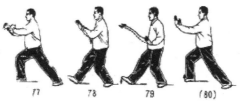

Sweep Left and Right to turn 180 degrees + 45 degrees more.

Form 9   **Step Out with Left Foot and Single Whip**

• Right hand sweeps to the right at head level and

becomes a bird's tail .

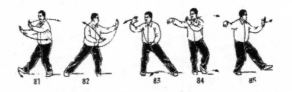

• Left hand moves down across body then waves up

past the face and pushes to left side as you turn the waist

and step left.

(Rock back. Turn to face front turning on left heel only.)

Form 10   **Wave Hands Like Clouds (3 times)**

• Left hand makes a downward arc across front of body,

then waves up past the face.

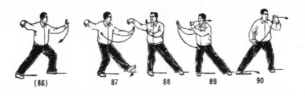

178

• Right foot drags in.

• Right hand moves across front of body, palm down

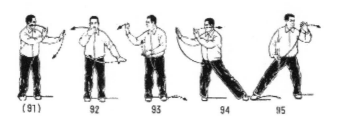

• Turn waist to left.

• Turn palms over, left hand descends, right hand rises and waves past the face as waist turns to right.

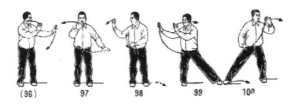

Step sideways with left foot, repeat twice more.

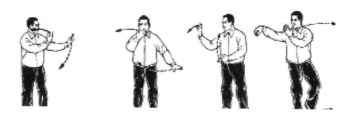

(Step on the diagonal with left foot to start next movement.)

Form 11   **Single Whip**

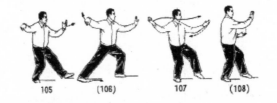

• As left foot steps, right hand becomes a bird's tail.

•Left hand rises, palm up, to wave past the face, then pushes forward, palm out.

(Drag right foot 1/2 step, shift weight to back foot.)

Form 12   **Pierce Cloud**

• Right hand descends, then rises, palm facing you.

• Cross hands as arms rise above head. Turn palms outward.

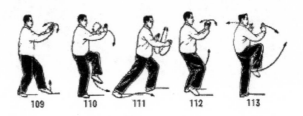

• Arms descend at sides as you bend over (gather down

• As you straighten up, cross hands in front of yourself.

(Left foot steps out on an angle.)

Form 13   Kick with Right Foot

• Separate hands at shoulder level: left hand to the side,

right arm over right leg for balance as you kick.

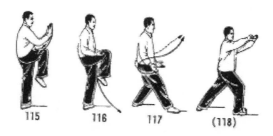

Form 14   Stroke the Beard/Double Wind Meets the Ears

• Palms turn in toward chest, backs of hands meet.

• Turn fingers up and then stroke downward with both

hands, separating them as they brush down across right

thigh.

• Put right foot down and rock forward while making an

upward circle with arms until knuckles of hands

(loose fist) almost meet in front at chest level.

(Rock back and turn, heel then toe, 180°)

Form 15   **Gather Down**

• After the turn, open the hands to the sides and downward, gathering in toward the body.

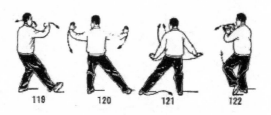

• As you straighten up, cross hands as if gathering into the chest. Then as you kick with left heel, uncross the hands.

• Hands separate for balance: left hand out over kicking left leg, right arm to the side.

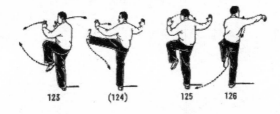

• Right hand becomes a bird's tail as left hand moves to right hip, palm up.

(Slide left leg out to the side, toes pointing to the left.)

Form 16   **Push Down and Stand On One Leg - Left Style**

(Snake Creeps Down)

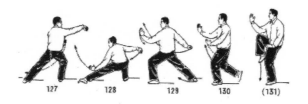

• Bend with head over right knee.

•As body turns to left, left hand pushes down inside of left leg

•Right hand moves to lower back, still in a bird's tail. Left knee bends.

• As you straighten up, putting weight on left leg, step forward with right foot. Right hand moves from behind to the front and hands come up in 7 Stars.

(Adjust left foot.)

Form 17   **Push Down and Stand On One Leg - Right Style**

(Snake Creeps Down)

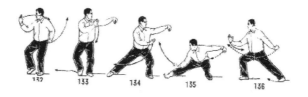

• Draw right foot into left instep, left hand makes a bird's tail.

• Bend with head over left knee.

• As body turns to right, right hand pushes down inside of right leg.

• Left hand moves to lower back, still in a bird's tail. Right knee bends.

• Straighten up, putting weight on right leg. Left hand comes from behind, hands come up in 7 Stars as left foot steps forward, twist step.

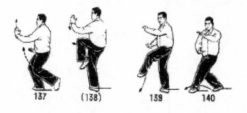

Form 18   **Fair Lady Looks in Mirror/Work Shuttles on Both Sides**

• As you step to the right, raise right hand as in 'raising single hand," press right hand to the right side. Left hand push the shuttle up, striking toward the jaw.

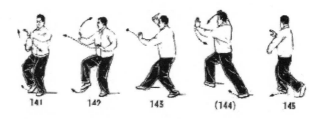

- Rock back, step to the left. Gather a ball and press to the left side. Left hand rising as in " raising single hand," right hand push the shuttle up, striking toward the jaw.

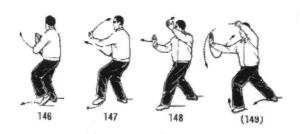

(Drag back foot 1/2 step. Shift weight back to elbow strike.)

Form 19   **Needle At the Sea Bottom**

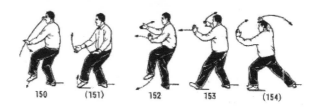

- Both hands move to center of torso, right hand higher

than the left. Fingers of left hand point out, fingers of right hand point down.

• Bend over as the right hand sinks to the ground to pick up the needle. Left hand does not move.

(Straighten up and step out with left foot.)

Form 20   Flash Arms

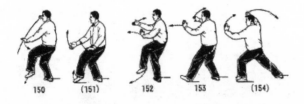

(Rock back.)

Form 21   Turn (180°) and Chop (knuckles down)

(Also called Deflect-Downward, Parry & Punch)

• Turn on left heel, then right toe 180°

• While turning, make a circle in front of the body with right arm. After pivoting on the right toe, step out with right foot and chop, knuckles down.

• Step forward with left foot as right hand makes a circle to right side, then punches over left wrist.

• Draw both hands back at waist, rocking back.

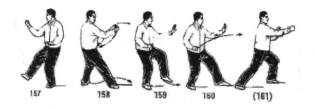

• Rock forward and press arms forward.

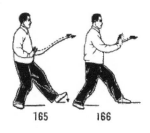

(Turn to right 1/4 turn.)

Form 22   **Apparent Close-up**

• Slide right foot out, keeping weight on the left, and gather down with right hand. Left pushes out to left, right hand pushes out to right as you straighten up.

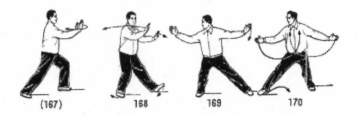

Form 23   Cross Hands
(Right foot slides in, then left foot steps out slightly.)

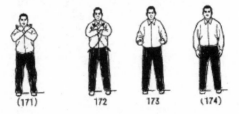

Form 24   Conclusion

• Collect the Qi - Make an upward circle with arms, palms down, wrists relaxed, as you breathe in draw up the yin Qi. When hands pass your heart turn them upward to gather the yang Qi. When hands are over your head turn palms towards the top of the head, the Bai Hui acupuncture point. Press down in front of the body as you breathe out, sending the Qi down to the dantian.. Repeat two more times.

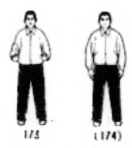

I/5   (I/4)

• After third time, push Qi into Dantian (1.6 inches

below the navel, inside the abdomen) by covering the

Dantian.

• Step back and make the traditional bow thanking your

teachers for teaching you.

Richard Leirer

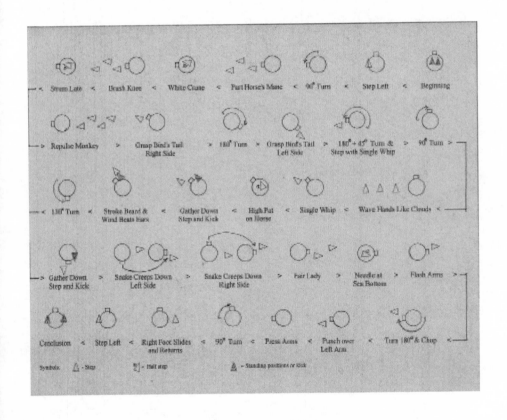

24 Tai Chi Stepping Diagram

Chapter Ten

Adult Stem Cell Production
Ancient Bone Marrow Washing Qigong
成人幹細胞生產＝古代骨髓洗衣機氣功

The future of Western medicine is in the regeneration of body parts to increase health and prolong healthy life. Stem Cells, particularly Adult Stem Cells, will provide the method for this future medicine. An Adult Stem Cell can become any body part. It has the ability to dedifferentiate into any and all cells within the body. These stem cells are found everywhere in the body and are produced in the bone marrow when new blood is produced. Some current therapies extract these stem cells from the blood or directly from the bone marrow of a client and then increase the number of cells by growing more in a lab setting. After growing more of the clients' own stem cells, those cells are then reinserted into the body at the site of damage or injury. Because a Stem Cell can become any other cell within the body, regeneration of the damaged or injured area occurs.

Adult stem cells are the Wu Chi of the body. Like Wu Chi, these cells contain all of the potential to become any cell.

Richard Leirer

On Monday September 24, 2007 at the 2007 Congress of Neurological Surgeons Annual Meeting in California, researchers announced preliminary results involving 38 Patients in a clinical trial that used the implantation of autologous adult bone marrow stem cells into spinal cord injury (SCI) patients – resulting in some restored function for patients who had been paralyzed for an average of four years, some up to twenty two years.

Dr. Luis Geffner presented a preliminary report at the 2007 Congress of Neurological Surgeons Annual Meeting in San Diego. From May 2006 to August 2007, 38 patients with SCI were treated at Luis Vernaza Hospital in Guayaquil, Ecuador. They were treated with autologous bone marrow stem cells – meaning the cells were extracted from the patients' own bone marrow, taken from the hip bone (iliac crests).

Of the 25 patients who provided more than three months and up to 14 months follow up: 15 gained the ability to stand up, 10 could walk on the parallels with braces, seven could walk without braces and five could walk with crutches. Three patients

192

recovered full bladder control, and 10 patients regained some form of sexual function. No adverse events or abnormal reactions to implantation were observed. (Geffner, Luis *Clinical Trial Suggests Bone Marrow Stem Cells Are Useful for Spinal Cord Injury* http://sci.rutgers.edu/forum/arChive/index.php/t-84242.html n.p.n.d. web 2012)

In other studies researchers found that adult stem cells can be used for many purposes without having to add to or change the cell.

Scientists at Children's Hospital of Pittsburgh of UPMC have discovered a unique population of adult stem cells derived from human muscle that could be used to treat muscle injuries and diseases such as heart attack and muscular dystrophy.

In a study using human muscle tissue, scientists in Children's Stem Cell Research Center - led by Johnny Huard, PhD, and Bruno Péault, PhD – isolated and characterized stem cells taken from blood vessels (known as myoendothelial cells) that are easily isolated using cell-sorting techniques that proliferate rapidly and can be differentiated in the laboratory into muscle, bone and cartilage cells.

The exciting aspect of this research is, our human body has the ability to make cells that can become anything in our body. The research indicates that these cells that are already in our body can go to a specific location in the body and then they do the job of becoming what needs to be repaired. These adult stem cells do not have to be changed or tweaked or modified. They are cells with the ability to become anything in the human body including a heart cell or a liver cell or a muscle cell, anything.

An ancient Qigong practice called Bone Marrow Washing recognized the importance of the bone marrow in stem cell production. The bone marrow is where the stem cells are created along with new blood cells for the body. These adult stem cells then travel through the body working to create any new tissue within the body. We can use the cells we all have in our own body to repair any damage that has occurred in any area of the body.

The key is, we have to get the cell to that spot that needs repair. That is where Tai Chi, Qigong, Bone Marrow Washing and DNA reprogramming meditations come into play. The nature of Qigong/Tai Chi and Bone Marrow Washing practices with inward and downward pressure on the flat bones in the body, helps increase stem cell production. Those flat bones of the body are the breastbone, the top of the hip or iliac crest, and the wing bone or scapula. The relaxed nature of Qigong/Tai Chi movements provides for an increase in blood circulation with stem cells to all body sites, particularly the inner organs. Qigong/Tai Chi is known as an internal exercise. As the mind focuses on each movement, neural stimulation of every area of the body occurs. This increases circulation of the stem cells and helps to take away waste byproducts of cellular activity.

DNA reprogramming meditation is a specific type of meditation designed to penetrate the bone marrow and infuse all the new blood cells with Qi energy. This practice activates the Adult Stem Cells and circulates those cells to the major organs. (See author's website to order this meditation cd.)

In the 5 th century C.E. Da Mo, the Bohdidarma, traveled to China from India. He taught monks at the Shaolin temple in China special bone marrow washing exercises that increased health and revitalization. This Qigong exercise also increases both the production and circulation of the stem cells. Chinese Medial Doctors quickly saw the benefits of these practices and have incorporated the knowledge Da Mo brought to China by emphasizing blood circulation and exercise for creation of the adult stem cell. Part of the deficiency or excess patterns in Chinese Medical diagnosis has to do with stem cells and the health of the body.

Even after these stem cells are created and sent to become a body part, modern research indicates it might take up to 21 days for those new cells to work. A recent study shows,

> In fact, certain important synaptic connections – the circuitry that allows the brain cells to talk to each other – do not appear until 21 days after the birth of the new cells, according to Charles Greer, professor of neurosurgery and neurobiology, and senior author of the study. In the meantime, other areas of the brain provide information to the new cells, preventing them from disturbing ongoing functions until the cells are mature. *"The Journal of Neuroscience* 27: 9951-9961 (October 2007)

So even though the cell is in place it takes time to make the total body/ mind/nerve connection.

The ancient Chinese knew about the constantly changing cells of the human body for centuries. Master Huang explained to me in the early 1970's that the human body is best explained with the analogy of a person standing in a river or creek or small body of moving water. Within the time it takes to clap your hands, and without moving, are you still in the same water? In one way yes, it is still the same river or creek. In another way no, because it is new water that is now present and the old water has past. So it is with the human body. Old cells that make up our body are dying and being replaced all the time. The cells that die off are removed through the veins and new cells are pumped into the cells by the arteries. An average cell may live for as little as ninety days or less. So, think of your body as only really being less then 100 days old, regardless of your age.

Qigong Tai Chi and How Exercise Helps Depression and Anxiety According to the Mayo Clinic

Exercise has long been touted as a way to maintain physical fitness and help prevent high blood pressure, diabetes and other diseases. With the knowledge our bodies are in constant state of change and repair a growing volume of research shows that exercise can also help improve symptoms of certain mental health conditions, including depression and anxiety. Exercise may also help prevent a relapse after treatment for depression or anxiety.

Research suggests that it may take at least 30 minutes of exercise a day for at least three to five days a week to significantly improve depression symptoms. But smaller amounts of activity – as little as 10 to 15 minutes at a time – can improve mood in the short term. "Small bouts of exercise may be a great way to get started if it's initially too hard to do more," Dr. Vickers-Douglas says.

> Scientists at Duke University Medical Center tested exercise against Zoloft, and found the ability of either – or a combination of the two – to reduce or eliminate symptoms were about the same. They found that exercise seemed to do a better job of keeping symptoms from coming back after the depression lifted. The patients in this study had been diagnosed with major depressive disorder. This report followed earlier research in which 156 adult volunteers had taken part in a four-month comparison of exercise, Zoloft or a combination. The exercise primarily consisted of brisk walking, stationary bike riding, or jogging for 30 minutes, plus a 10-minute warm-up and 5-minute cool-down, three times a week.

Still another study published in the journal Psychosomatic Medicine, included 202 men and women age 40 and older who were diagnosed with major depression. They were randomly assigned to one of four groups: one that worked out in a supervised, group setting three times per week; one that exercised at home; one that took the antidepressant sertraline (Zoloft); and one that took placebo pills.

After 16 weeks, the patients completed standard measures of depression symptoms. By the end of the study, Blumenthal's team found, 47 percent of patients on the antidepressant no longer met the criteria for major depression. The same was true of 45 percent of those in the supervised exercise group.

In the home-based exercise group, 40 percent had their symptoms go into remission. That compared with 31 percent of the placebo group.

Swedish researchers say they may know why these health results occur. Research indicates that exercise stimulates the production of new brain cells.

In a series of studies by Astrid Bjornebekk at the Karolinska Institute have shown that both exercise and antidepressants help rats form new cells in the hippocampus, a part of the brain associated in humans with memory and learning.

However, a lecturer in Health Care Ethics at the School of Nursing in Dublin City University, Ireland says, ". . . . evidence there is suggests that the benefits of Tai Chi extend beyond those of simply exercising. It appears the combination of exercise, meditation, and breathing all help relieve anxiety and depression."

Other research shows how stress takes its toll on the body. Remember, Tai Chi reduces stress.

The National Institute of Mental Health reports that the stress hormones found in depressed women caused bone loss that gave them bones of women nearly twice their age.

Exactly why Tai Chi offers such benefits for women may be explained by a study from Australia's La Trobe University that found that Tai Chi reduced levels of stress hormones more effectively than some other forms of activity. Less stress, less bone loss.

Another study revealed that sex hormone levels may be balanced by the practice of Qigong exercises because female sex hormone (estrogen) levels tend to increase in men and decrease in women naturally.

Three studies indicate that Qigong exercise can reverse this trend. The effect of Qigong exercise on plasma sex hormone levels was determined for hypertensive men and women. The sex hormones levels were measured before and after Qigong practice for one year.

Results showed that high estrodiol levels in men lowered to near normal, and low estrodial levels in women raised to near normal after Qigong practice.

The science behind these reports testifies to the multiple health benefits of Qigong Tai Chi. (See appendix for study details.)

Harvard Health Publications, in May 2009, says "Tai Chi is often described as 'meditation in motion,' but it might well be called '*medication in motion*.' There is growing evidence that this mind-body practice, which originated in China as a martial art, has value in treating or preventing many health problems.

And you can get started even if you aren't in top shape or the best of health. 'A growing body of carefully conducted research is building a compelling case for Tai Chi as an adjunct to standard medical treatment for the prevention and rehabilitation of many conditions commonly associated with age,' says Peter M. Wayne, assistant professor of medicine at Harvard Medical School and director of the Tai Chi and Mind-Body Research Program at Harvard Medical School's Osher Research Center. An adjunct therapy is one that's used together with primary medical treatments, either to address a disease itself or its primary symptoms, or, more generally, to improve a patient's functioning and quality of life."

"No pain, big gains."

Although Tai Chi is slow and gentle and doesn't leave you breathless, it addresses the key components of fitness, including muscle strength, flexibility, balance, and, to a lesser degree, aerobic conditioning. Here's some of the evidence:

Muscle Strength. In a 2006 study published in *Alternative Therapies in Health and Medicine,* Stanford University researchers reported benefits of tai Chi in 39 women and men, average age 66, with below-average fitness and at least one cardiovascular risk factor. After taking 36 tai Chi classes in 12 weeks, they showed improvement in both lower-body strength (measured by the number of times they could rise from a chair in 30 seconds) and upper-body strength (measured by their ability to do arm curls).

In a Japanese study using the same strength measures, 113 older adults were assigned to different 12-week exercise programs, including Tai Chi, brisk walking, and resistance training. People who did Tai Chi improved more than 30% in lower-body strength and 25% in arm strength – almost as much as those who participated in resistance training, and more than those assigned to brisk walking.

Internist Dr. Gloria Yeh, an assistant professor at Harvard Medical School says, "Although you aren't working with weights or resistance bands, the unsupported arm exercise involved in Tai Chi strengthens your upper body." She added, "Tai Chi strengthens both the lower and upper extremities and also the core muscles of the back and abdomen."

Flexibility:

Women in the 2006 Stanford study significantly boosted upper and lower-body flexibility as well as strength.

Balance:

Tai Chi improves balance and, according to some studies, reduces falls. Proprioception, which is the ability to sense the position of one's body in space declines with age. Tai Chi helps train this sense, which is a function of sensory neurons in the inner ear and stretch receptors in the muscles and ligaments. Tai Chi also improves muscle strength and flexibility, which makes it easier to recover from a stumble. Fear of falling can make you more likely to fall; some studies have found that tai Chi training helps reduce that fear.

Aerobic Conditioning:

Tai Chi is also more aerobic than aerobic exercise conditioning. Tai Chi delivers more oxygen to the blood through greater circulation and deeper breathing then aerobic exercise. In aerobic exercise a person decreases the oxygen supply, tenses muscles, reducing circulation and oxygen deliver to the cell. There is also an increase in uric acid in aerobic conditioning that does not occur with Tai Chi and Qigong. High uric acid leads to gout or potential kidney disease. Tai Chi and Qigong help the body.

The ancient Chinese sages and doctors knew how important stem cells are to the human body. They did not have the same name for it, but knew its function. They also knew Qigong and Tai Chi increase those stem cell production and circulation through out the body creating a strong and healthy body. Tai Chi and Qigong are proven to be full of ancient wisdom for a modern world.

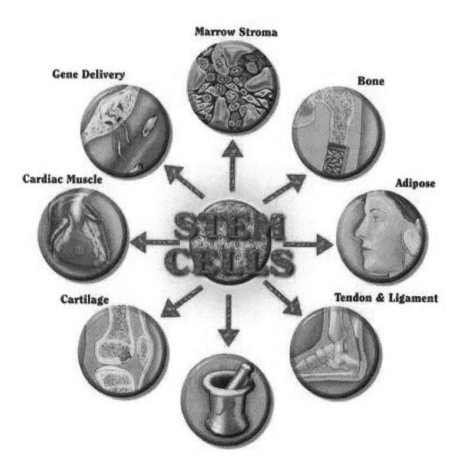

Picture courtesy of Imgur

Final Notes

There is an ancient Chinese saying, One hundred days to build the foundation, ten months to produce the embryo and three years to baby-sit. This is the process of the gradual growth of our expanding consciousness. Ken Wilber aptly calls the results of this growth "*The Spectrum of Consciousness*" and his book by that title is considered a classic in transpersonal psychology. The ancient Chinese understood this and created techniques for awareness and consciousness training.

This is a first of three writings I have planned to help the reader facilitate that growth. *From Wu Chi to Tai Chi: A story of Ancient Beginnings* sets the backdrop and gives us ample thought and considerable energy work to cultivate.

The second writing, *Ten Months to Produce the Embryo*, will deal with a program of Nei Gong or internal Qigong energy work that will reveal the inner alchemy needed to progress to a more fuller awakening.

The third writing , *Three years to Babysit,* will give practical advice on how to live in a new world with an expanded level of consciousness.

It can be enough to just practice the works outlined in this book. If you practice, you will reap the rewards. From my personal experience I can tell you that I learned the movements outlined here in a very short period of time. That is unusual. The average person takes from 3-5 years to learn a form. However I was dedicated and young, only 18 yrs old when I began. I wanted to learn the movements and techniques. I practiced four to five times a day. I practiced in the morning before work, in my morning break at work, at lunchtime, in my afternoon break and sometime in the evening before bed. I was dedicated to learning and practicing. Having learned the forms I was able to practice and perform on my own. Yet each and every time I practiced in a group at class, I felt different. I felt happier and more Qi-filled. It was noticeable and palpable to me. Years went by and I continued my practice, still recognizing a major difference in Qi feelings and in my own personal sense of well being that was heightened in a class setting. The class settings were not all that interesting to me any longer. I had already learned the forms and was somewhat bored with having heard the same hing over and over again as way of an explanation. I had been practicing for over 10 years.

Still, I recognized the difference when I practiced alone or with the group in a class. So one day I approached my teacher, Lee Henn. I said, "Lee there is a great noticeable difference in my Tai Chi practice when I am alone and when I am in a group. Why is that?" My teacher looked at me and smiled and said, "Richard, you know the answer to that." I said I did not. My teacher smiled again and said, "yes you do." I became angry and said very sternly "Don't give me any of that metaphysical bullshit. I want to know." Again, just a smile in return. In anger I stomped out of the classroom, boiling and muttering to myself, " Stupid answer."

I went home and stewed for a long time. Weeks went by, and I was still angry. I set my mind to find the answer myself. What were the variables that changed between my practice by myself or in a group? The answer was not hard to discover. That variable I was looking for was simple. That variable was other people. Other people, whether they were skilled or unskilled in Tai Chi, made the difference in what I experienced. They made a difference that I could easily recognize and one I could feel.

How was this possible? How can such a thing be true? I was raised in the United States from strong Austrian /German and Polish ancestry home. I was taught to be self reliant and hard working. I was also taught to not rely on others.

Now my whole vision of the world came crashing down on me. The paradigm I had shaped my life around was proving itself to be not as effective as I was led to believe. People, ordinary people, are important to me. This was a major shock for me. How could this be true? Everyday people, not just the selected individuals I had let into my life, held an importance to my quality of life. What a shock and what an awakening for me. It is for this reason we call practicing Qigong Tai Chi " Playing." We play Tai Chi together. We grow together and we can awaken together.

The *Course in Miracles* reminds us:

" Everyone you do meet you are to meet for your mutual awakening."

Master Hao Tien You tried to explain this to me in during my Qigong training with the following story.

> There once was a young monk who was told to hurry to the well and fetch a jar of water for his Master. He was instructed not to tarry and not to waste his time talking to strangers. He was to hurry and bring the water back for the Master. So off the young monk goes to the river to fill the jug. Filling the jug, and

hurrying back he sees and old woman who kindly asks him for a little water. He remembers that his Master told him to not delay and to not talk to anyone on the way. He says to the old woman, " This water is for my Master, I cannot give any to you." Off he goes back to the Master. Upon his arrival the Master says to the young monk. "How did it go?" "Oh it went well," was the reply. "Did anything unusual happen on your journey?" the master asked. "Oh no said the young monk." " Are you sure," asked the Master. "Of course I am sure. I went to the river as you instructed and I raced back here as fast as I could without delay." "Tell me all that you saw and all that you did," said the Master. Again repeating what was already told, the young monk paused after explaining how he got to the river and then he remembered the old woman. He told the Master, "Oh yes, there was an old woman who stopped me and asked for water. I told her the water was for you and I hurried back here as instructed." Upon hearing this new information about the old woman the old master said, "Ohh, you poor monk. Do you realize what you have done?" "No," came the reply. "You missed the Great Master," said the Master monk. " What Great Master?" asked the young monk. "The old woman," he replied. "How is she the Great Master?" asked the young monk. "Oh, the masters disguise themselves in many ways. Appearances are always deceiving. Look with your heart and not your eyes and you will be able to see," was the answer.

Richard Leirer

Appendix

Benefits of Qigong and Tai Chi on Health and Healing
Written by Shin Lin, Ph.D.

In Theses: Scientific and Skill Papers on Qigong, published in coordination with The World Qigong Forum 2007 and 10th World Congress on Qigong and Traditional Chinese Medicine, Tokyo, 2007, p.3-8.

Research Leading to a Systems/Cellular/Molecular Model for the Benefits of Qigong and Tai Chi on Health and Healing

Shin LIN

Laboratory for Mind-Body Signaling & Energy Research and Susan Samueli Center for Integrative Medicine, University of California (Irvine, USA)

Abstract: The goal of our research is to apply modern biomedical technologies to develop experimental approaches, protocols, and instrumentation, and use them to quantify physiological and bioenergetics changes associated with the practice of Qigong and Tai Chi. In our studies on dozens of high level practitioners and many control subjects over the last few years, we have shown that Qigong and Tai Chi (a) increase blood flow measured by laser Doppler flowmetry, (b) induce a state of relaxation as indicated by heart rate variability analysis of electroencephalography and brain wave analysis of electroencephalography, and (c) elevate bioenergy emission in the form of heat (infrared thermography), light (single photon counting), electrical charge (gas discharge visualization), and conductance at acupuncture points (pre-polarization measurement with single square voltage). Based these results and previous studies by other investigators, we propose a working model for explaining the many effects of Qigong and Tai Chi on health and healing at the systems, cellular, and molecular levels. We hope that our on-going experiments and this model will stimulate future research that leads to a better understanding of the scientific basis of the these practices and thus accelerate their integration into the global healthcare community.

Keywords: Qigong, Tai Chi, Physiology, Bioenergy, Health and Healing, Systems-Cellular-Molecular Model

1. Introduction

The many different styles and schools of Chinese mind/body practices involving regulation of mind, body, and respiration (i.e., Qigong and Tai Chi), are traditionally thought to enhance health and healing by improving the level and circulation of "Qi", the Chinese term for vital energy (1-3). Because Qi is an ancient concept that does not have a precise scientific definition (2), the goal of research in our laboratory is to apply modern biomedical technologies to develop experimental approaches,

protocols, and instrumentation, and use them to quantify physiological and bioenergetic changes associated with the practice of Qigong and Tai Chi. This paper summarizes our progress and presents a model based on our studies and those of others to explain the major benefits of Qigong and Tai Chi at the systems, cellular, and molecular levels. We hope that our work and this model will stimulate future research that leads to a better understanding of the scientific basis of the these practices and thus accelerate their integration into the global healthcare community.

2. Physiological Changes Associated with Qigong and Tai Chi Practices

There is a considerable volume of literature documenting how Tai Chi as a physical exercise can improve musculoskeletal parameters such as body flexibility and balance (4-6). Other studies have shown that Tai Chi and Qigong practices can improve indicators of health such as blood pressure, lipid profile, self-report of stress reduction, and immune markers (5-9). In this part of our studies, we focused on the effects of Qigong and Tai Chi on the nervous system and the cardiovascular system. The following is a summary of results obtained from on-going studies involving several dozen high-level practitioners as well as many control subjects.

a. Effects on the Autonomic Nervous System.

Heart rate variability (HRV) analysis of data from electrocardiography (EKG) is becoming an increasingly common method to non-invasively evaluate autonomic nervous function. In many studies, low frequency variability (LF, < 0.15 Hz as shown in the power spectrum produced by fast Fourier transformation of time series data) is taken as an indicator of sympathetic tone, and high frequency variability (HF, > 0.15 Hz) as an indicator of parasympathetic tone (10). To examine how HRV can be applied to the study of physiological changes associated with mind/body practices, we used a portable Holter system designed by our collaborator Dr. Zhong-Yuan Shen of the Qigong Research Institute at the Shanghai University of Traditional Chinese Medicine. The system has the capability of simultaneous recording of EKG and respiratory pattern measured with chest and abdominal straps containing stretch transducers.

Based on studies on over a dozen Qigong and Tai Chi practitioners and 20+ control subjects, we determined that a number of factors can significantly influence HRV (11). First, the frequency of the breathing cycle influences the frequency of the HRV peak produced by a mechanism referred to as respiratory sinus arrhythmia (RSA). Thus, a practitioner with a heart rate of 60 beats per minute will produce a HF peak at 0.2 Hz by regulating breathing at the rate of 12 cycles per minute, and a LF peak at 0.1 Hz when the breathing rate is slowed down to 6 cycles per minute. This shift from HF to LF is not necessarily a reflection of a change from a state of relaxation to a state of stress (i.e. higher parasympathetic to higher sympathetic function) as previously stated (10). Furthermore, multiple HF peaks may be produced by breathing at different rates during the measurement period (e.g., 3 different peaks produced by breathing at 8, 12, and 16 cycles per minute at different time intervals), thereby complicating the analysis of the power spectrum. On the other hand, we have also found in some cases involving younger subjects what appeared to be harmonics at higher frequencies even though they were strictly controlling their breathing at a single rate throughout the measurement period. For example, a subject in his early twenties breathing at a steady rate of 6 cycles per minutes (0.1 Hz) could still produce peaks at 0.2, 0.3, 0.4 Hz, etc., with diminishing amplitude in both the power spectra of the HRV and of the breathing pattern.

Second, the size of the HRV peak produced by RSA is dependent not just on the tidal volume of each breath, but also on the posture of the subject. For instance, a subject breathing at a controlled rate and volume will show a larger peak in the sitting position compared to the standing position, and an even larger peak in the supine position. Therefore, it is difficult to directly compare the HRV of a given subject practicing meditation in the sitting position and in the standing position. On the other hand, it is important that for those subjects who were in the sitting position throughout the experiment, their HF peak tended to increase in size during meditation compared to the periods before and after the practice (12,13). Because a high HF peak was also seen during a period of deep sleep in control subjects, this result supports the notion that meditation is a very effective way to reach a state of rest and relaxation.

Third, under the same conditions, younger subjects (20-25 year olds in this study) generally show a larger peak produced by RSA compared to older subjects (50-70 year old). This effect sometimes overshadows differences based on other considerations, such as years of training in mind-body practices.

In conclusion, this part of our study shows that HRV analysis can be a useful tool for assessing autonomic nervous function in mind/body practices (13), but great care must be taken to control all of the factors indicated above.

b. Effects on Brain Function.

Pilot experiments involving electroencephalography (EEG) were conducted in collaboration with Dr. Ramesh Srinivasan at the Cognitive Science Department of University of California, Irvine, and with Dr. Tzyy-Ping Jung at the Swartz Center for Computational Neuroscience of the University of California, San Diego (12). A number of experienced Qigong and Tai Chi practitioners were recorded with a 128-channel EEG system (Geodesic Sensor Net System from Electrical Geodesic, Inc.) before, during, and after meditation in the sitting position. With highly experienced subjects, there was an increase in alpha and theta waves recorded at the frontal mid-line area of the head within minutes into the meditative period compared to the baseline level recorded before and after this period. When the EEG data were further examined by the method of Independent Component Analysis (14), we found that the increase in alpha and theta waves was also accompanied by an increase in beta waves (12,13). Since alpha and theta waves signify a state of relaxation and rest while beta waves reflect a state of alert consciousness, this analysis indicates that meditation is a dual state of "relaxed concentration". This conclusion is consistent with the commonly held notion that mediation is not only an excellent means to aChieve deep rest, but also an effective way to train the mind to be sharply focused during mental activities in every day life.

c. Effects on the Circulatory System.

In Traditional Chinese Medicine, the close relationship between blood flow and Qi is illustrated by the common sayings "blood is the mother of Qi" and "when intention comes, so comes the Qi, and so comes the blood". In this part of our studies, peripheral blood flow was measured by laser Doppler flowmetry (15) at the skin level (i.e., cutaneous blood flow) by placing a probe of the instrument (Model DRT4 from Moor Instruments, Ltd.) on the Lao Gong (PC8) acupuncture point (acupoint) on the palm.

A dozen subjects were instructed to perform the single-handed silk-reeling exercise of Chen Style Tai Chi, which consists of a slow, repetitive, elongated circular movement of the right arm and an up-and-down movement of the legs, all coordinated with deep breathing cycles at the rate of about 4 times per minute. This type of exercise, as well as some other Tai Chi and Qigong movements, were found to increase the "flux" of blood flow (i.e., speed multiply by the number of red cells within the volume of tissue measured) measured at the moving hand by ~50-300%. In general, this increase in blood flow was primarily due to the arm movement. The coordinated leg movement and deep breathing cycles were also contributors to this effect, but the degree of their effects varied from subject to subject. In general, the overall effect of Qigong and Tai Chi practice on blood flow tends to be greater when the subject is more experienced and more mentally and physically relaxed.

To have a better understanding of the effect of breathing regulation on blood flow, we made simultaneous recordings of EKG, breathing pattern, and blood flow on subjects during deep breathing cycles. It was apparent from the analysis of the combined data that the increase in instantaneous heart rate (measured as time interval between two beats) caused by the slow, deep inhalation phase (i.e., RSA as described in Section IIA) led to increased blood flow (16). Thus, proper coupling of deep breathing cycles with certain Qigong and Tai Chi movements can further increase blood flow as described above. In general, the combined effect tends to be greater for more experienced subjects.

3. Bioenergetic Changes Associated with Qigong and Tai Chi Practices

In Traditional Chinese Medicine, the healing effects of Qigong are often explained as enhancement of the level and flow of Qi. Western biomedical research on these two types of interventions has been hampered by the lack of a strict scientific definition of Qi, which is based more on human feelings and experiences rather than the physicist's definitions of energy, force, fields, etc. (2). One approach around this dilemma is to study those changes in energy that are measurable with modern instrumentation. Our studies to date have indicated that Qigong and Tai Chi practices do produce a number of measurable energy-related changes.

a. Effects on Electrical Conductance at Acupoints.

The "Single Square Voltage Pulse" (SSVP) method was developed by Motoyama to measure conductance before polarization (BP) and after polarization (AP) at jing-

well acupoints (17). He proposed that BP is an indication of the bioenergy of the corresponding meridians while AP is related to stress commonly measured as galvanic skin response (17,18). Besides measuring the conductance values with a 1 millisecond pulse of 3 volts rather than with a constant current, the method also incorporates the use of a hand-held electrode probe with a flexible shank to make electrical contact with an adhesive sponge electrode pad pre-placed on the acupoint, a method designed to minimize physical stimulation of the acupoint by the probe during the measurement.

We conducted a detailed examination of the variability of the SSVP instrumentation (AMI Care System from AMICA Co., Japan) and methodology under different conditions (19). First, by using a micromanipulator (Model M from Leitz Corp., Germany) to place the electrode probe onto an electrode pad adhered to the jing-well acupoint of the Pericardium Meridian on the hand, we showed that the average variability values of the BP and AP measurements were 0.6% and 2.0%, respectively, based on 165 sets of 27 continuous measurements on 6 subjects made without lifting the probe off the electrode pad. These values represent the minimum aChievable reproducibility of the SSVP method under idealized conditions. Furthermore, we found that increasing the pressure of the probe on the electrode pad by adjusting the setting on the micromanipulator resulted in an increase of the BP value by 3-5%, with occasionally a slight increase in variability. Under normal experimental conditions when the probe was placed by hand on electrode pads on all 28 jing-well acupoints on the hands and feet of 5 subjects, the variability was 8 % for BP and 15% for AP, based on 10 rounds of measurements with the same set of pads.

Appendix

How mind-body exercises might affect BP and AP values was investigated in our study involving measurement of 9 advanced subjects (3 of them measured twice) with an average of 23 years of experience before and after 15-20 minutes of Tai Chi practice (13,16). We found that in all cases, there was an increase of overall BP (average of BP measured at the 28 jing-well acupoints) ranging from 8-26 % (average of 17%). In related experiments involving some of these subjects as well as other control subjects, riding a stationary bicycle and lifting weights produce little or no effect on BP values. Compared to BP, we did not find a definitive pattern of change with respect to overall AP values in subjects practicing Tai Chi in this study (6 cases increased, 4 cases decreased, and 2 cases showed no change).

In conclusion, this part of our studies shows that the SSVP method has a low level of variability particularly when the difference in pressure exerted by the electrode probe on the conducting electrode pad is minimized. The study on Tai Chi practitioners indicates that BP values can be a useful marker for studying the bioenergetic effects of mind-body practices.

b. Effects on Biophoton Emission.

The human body is known to emit a low level of energy in the form of light in the visible range of the spectrum. This form of energy is referred to as biophotons (20). In this part of our studies, we assembled a system that can quantify biophoton emission from the palm of the hand with sensitivity at the level of a single photon (21). The instrumentation consists of a photomultiplier tube sensitive to light of ~300-600 nm (Integrated Counting Head, Model H59020-01 from Hamamatsu Corp., powered by Linear Power Supply, Model LPS-304/CE, from AMREL), connected to a timer/counter/analyzer (Model PM6680B/016, from Fluke), which sends the information to a standard desktop computer for analysis with the TimeView software. The photomultiplier tube, mounted on a stable frame to guide the placement of the hand, is housed inside a lightproof chamber with a sleeve for insertion of the hand.

We determined that a number of parameters must be precisely controlled in order to produce reliable data with our single photon counting system (21). First, while the background noise of the photomultiplier tube is sufficiently low and constant for this type of application ("dark counts" obtained in the absence of the hand are about 10 counts per second), it goes up rapidly when the temperature of the tube rises above 25o C. Thus cooling of the tube with a coil containing circulating water of a set temperature is essential to its proper operation. Second, the photon count decreases steadily with distance of the hand from the photomultiplier tube. Third, biophoton emission is highest at the center of the palm (i.e., around the Lao Gong, PC8, acupoint), and decreases towards the fingertips. Fourth, exposure of the hand to direct sunlight for even a few minutes can increase biophoton emission by 100 times or more for a couple of hours. Normal indoor lighting has relatively small effect on biophoton emission unless a subject's hand is within a few feet from a light bulb. Fifth, body temperature is another important factor affecting biophoton emission. In a study involving 10 control subjects, warming the hand to increase its temperature by 3o C increased biophoton emission by about 15% while cooling the hand by 14o C resulted in a similar level of change in the opposite direction. By carefully controlling all of the factors described above, we can aChieve a low variability of around 2-5% in our biophoton measurements.

Our single photon counting system was used to investigate the effect of different types of exercises on biophoton emission (21). First, 7 subjects were instructed to ride a stationary bicycle with hand and foot pedals (Airdyne from Schwinn) at a comfortable speed of around 60 cycles/minute for 15 minutes. Afterwards, 6 of the subjects showed an average increase in biophoton emission of 45% while one showed no change. Second, 12 subjects with no previous Tai Chi experience were instructed to perform the "silk reeling" movement of Chen style Tai Chi for 15 minutes. Afterwards, 11 of the subjects showed an average increase in biophoton emission of about 15% while one subject showed no significant change. As indicated below, a highly trained Tai Chi practitioner produced a higher level of change, but more experiments must be done to see whether this difference is statistically significant. In any case, this preliminary study shows that with careful control of the factors described above, the single photon counting system can produce useful data on the effect of exercises on bioenergy emission in the form of visible light.

c. Comparison Between Mind-Body and Physical Exercises.

Our ongoing studies have indicated that Tai Chi and Qigong can increase bioenergy measured as electrical conductance and biophoton emission (13,16,19, 21). To distinguish the effects of mind-body exercises from physical exercises, we directly compared 20 minutes of practice of the slow-soft movements from Old Frame Routine 1 of Chen Style Tai Chi (from which Yang Style Tai Chi was derived) with the relatively fast-hard movements from Routine 2 (similar to those of many 'hard" Kung Fu styles) (22). The subject in this pilot experiment was one of the top leaders of Chen Style Tai Chi from the Chen Family Village in China (birthplace of Tai Chi), who has more than 40 years of training in this type of practice. The effects of Routine 1 and Routine 2 were measured separately on two consecutive days. At least three sets of measurements were made with each instrument for each condition and the results were presented as averages.

First, the fast and hard movements of Routine 2 increased heart rate about twice as much as Routine 1 movements, reflecting the fact that it is a more vigorous physical activity. Second, the slow and soft movements of Routine 1 compared to Routine 2 movements produced a greater increase in pre-polarization electrical conductance at 28 jing-well acupoints measured with the Motoyama's single square voltage pulse

Appendix

method (18% vs 8% for hand acupoints and 42% vs 31% for foot acupoints), consistent with our previous observation that Tai Chi and Qigong can produce a bigger increase in this type of measurements compared with physical exercises such as riding a stationary bicycle and lifting weights (16). Third, the Routine 1 movements produced a greater increase in biophoton emission measured with the single photon counting system (55% vs 15%). Finally, the Routine 1 movements also produced a higher level of heat emission measured at the palm with infrared thermography (increase of 1.0 oC vs 0.6 oC), as well as a greater change in bioelectrical charge measured at the 10 finger tips with the method of gas discharge visualization (23) (+7% vs –4 % in average area of discharge pattern of all finger tips). The results of this case study indicate that for a top level Tai Chi practitioner, the slow and soft mind-body type of movements produced a greater change in all of the bioenergy markers measured compared to the more physical type of movements.

d. Effect on Physical Strength.

We wanted to see if the increase in bioenergy measured as heat, light, and electrical parameters produced by Tai Chi practice could also be measured in terms of physical strength. In a pilot study involving 5 subjects, the maximum weight they could lift a single time (referred to in weight training as 1-Rep Max) in a standardized test with a Bowflex maChine was calculated as previously described (24). For each subject, the measurement was made on one day and repeated on a different day after practicing 15 minutes of Tai Chi silk reeling movements. We found that all 5 subjects were able to lift an average of 10% more weight when the measurements were made following the Tai Chi practice. This level of increased strength is roughly equivalent to the gain from a few weeks of weight training in the absence of any Tai Chi practice. Thus, it appears that the bioenergy increase produce by Tai Chi practice can also be measured as an increase in physical strength.

e. Relationship between Blood Flow and Bioenergy.

The studies described above indicate that Tai Chi and Qigong practices can increase both blood flow and bioenergy markers, consistent with the Chinese concept of "blood is the mother of Qi". This relationship was further investigated in experiments in which blood flow was artificially increased by elevating the temperature of the hand by immersion in ~40oC water for 1-3 minutes (25). This treatment, which increased the temperature of the hand measured by infrared thermography by 3oC, produced similar increases in biophoton emission and pre-polarization conductance at acupoints at the hand as practicing Qigong and Tai Chi. Reducing the temperature of the hand by 140C by immersion in iced water for about a minute produced opposite effects.

In a related experiment, blood flow was artificially increased by pushing the head of an electrical percussion massage instrument (Thumper Mini Pro, from Sharper Image) against the palm of the hand for 1-5 minutes to simulate the self-massage movements of some types of Qigong practice (25). This treatment also increased the bioenergy markers in a manner similar to warming up the hand.

In conclusion, these two experiments indicate that increased blood flow correlates with elevation of bioenergy markers, consistent with the traditional concept of a close relationship between blood and Qi. The biological mechanisms by which these parameters are related remain to be determined.

4. A Model for Explaining the Benefits of Qigong and Tai Chi

Based on our studies and on previous work by other investigators, a model for the myriad of healthful benefits of Qigong and Tai Chi practices on mind-body functions can be presented at the systems, cellular, and molecular levels.

a. Improvement of Physical and Metabolic Markers.

There is abundant evidence that Tai Chi can improve musculoskeletal parameters such as body flexibility, muscle strength, and balance (4-6). The latter effect is a result of Tai Chi's emphasis on moving the entire body as a single unit and the deliberate placement and shifting of body weight for maximum stability. The increase in body balance with this type of training translates into a reduction of falls (26), a important outcome particularly for the health and well-being of the elderly.

There are other studies showing that Tai Chi and Qigong practices improve health indicators such as blood pressure and lipid profile (7,8), benefits that can also be derived from various forms of physical exercises. A recent study found that Tai Chi also lowers the diabetic indicator hemoglobin A1c (27), supporting the common belief that it is an excellent activity for diabetic patients. This effect can be explained by previous research showing that contraction of muscles can stimulate secretion of interleukin-6 from this tissue (28). This type of cytokine accelerates breakdown of stored fat (lipolysis) and increases insulin sensitivity in the body, but at higher levels also enhances the inhibitory action of cortisol on the immune system (29). As a mild form of physical exercise, Tai Chi can stimulate secretion of interleukin-6 from muscle tissues to produce beneficial effects on lipid and sugar metabolism, but not reaChing a high enough level to inhibit the immune system compared to more vigorous physical activities such as riding a bicycle at full speed for an extended period of time (28).

The practice of repetitive movements of Qigong and Tai Chi (e.g., silk reeling exercises in Chen style Tai Chi and hand-guided deep breathing exercises referred to as "pulling air" in Wu Dang Qigong) can have additional benefits on many other physiological functions. Studies on cats have demonstrated that repetitive movements

Appendix

(i.e., grooming) can lead to a several fold increase in the activity of serotonin neurons in the brain (30). These neurons connect widely with many parts of the brain and regulate directly or indirectly diverse physiological functions, including control of mood and emotion, sleep, digestion, cardiovascular and mental activities. Thus one could extrapolate from the animal studies that many of the beneficial effects of Qigong and Tai Chi could conceivably stem from the repetitive movements in these exercises.

b. Enhancement of Blood Flow.

It is common knowledge that physical exercises increase blood flow, particularly in the body directly involved in the activity. If the exercise is strenuous (lifting heavy weights), it becomes a stress to the body, inducing an increase in the tone of the sympathetic branch and a decrease of tone of the parasympathetic branch of the autonomic nervous system (31). This shift in autonomic balance leads to vasoconstriction all over the body except at the muscles directly involved (e.g., the biceps braChii in "biceps curl"). Qigong and Tai Chi movements, on the other hand, tend to be soft and slow and involve all parts of the body. Therefore, the effect is an increase in blood flow all over the body, particularly when the practitioner is in a relaxed mental and physical state and therefore high in parasympathetic tone. While this has not yet been a focus of our studies to date, results from pilot experiments with laser Doppler flowmetry are consistent with this notion.

The multi-functional Holter monitor system for simultaneous recording of EKG and breathing pattern allowed us to gain a better understanding of how the slow and deep breathing cycles in Qigong and Tai Chi can lead to an increase in heart rate and cardiac output. This phenomenon is mediated by the physiological mechanism referred to as respiratory sinus arrhythmia, which has previously been shown to be mediated mainly by the autonomic nervous system (32). Furthermore, by coupling the use of the Holter system with laser Doppler flowmetry, we can see how the effect of deep breathing cycles can add to the increase in blood flow due to Qigong and Tai Chi movements.

In conclusion, we can see how the essential elements of regulation of body, breath, and mind in Qigong and Tai Chi practices can contribute to enhancement of health and healing by increasing the transport of oxygen, nutrients, signaling factors, and waste materials by elevating blood flow all over the body.

c. Inducement of Relaxation

It is well recognized that a major reason mental stress is a serious detriment to good health is because of its inhibitory effect on the immune system, an action mediated by the stress hormone cortisol (33). In contrast, relaxation leads to a lowered sympathetic tone and subsequent decrease in cortisol secretion by the adrenal glands. In a pilot study, subjects who practiced Guolin Qigong (designed for cancer patients with emphasis on regulated breathing coordinated with a special style of walking) for 14 weeks had 20% lower cortisol and higher number of white blood cells secreting certain cytokines compared to the time when they started their training (9).

Another study showed that practicing an exercise derived from Tai Chi measurably increased cell mediated immunity (34). Consistent with that study, our analysis of heart rate variability and brain wave patterns in preliminary experiments indicated that Qigong meditation in the classical sitting position induced a state of relaxation. These findings are consistent with previous studies on other types of meditation (35,36). In collaboration with Dr. Zhong Yuan Shen of the Qigong Research Institute of the Shanghai University of Traditional Chinese Medicine, we are in the process of testing more advanced Holter monitors that are capable of simultaneous recordings of not just EKG and respiratory function, but also EEG and electromyography (EMG). This system should be valuable for more in depth studies on the "moving meditation" aspects of Tai Chi and Qigong practices in the future.

In conclusion, Qigong and Tai Chi are similar to many other types of mind-body practices in terms of inducing relaxation and relieving stress. By decreasing sympathetic function and increasing parasympathetic function of the autonomic nervous system, Qigong and Tai Chi can reverse stress-related effects such as inhibition of the immune system and poor blood circulation due to vasoconstriction.

d. Elevation of Bioenergy

Our single photon counting system for measuring light emission from the body proved to be a useful method for evaluating bioenergy changes associated with mind-body exercises. We used this instrument in combination with the more established technologies of laser Doppler flowmetry, gas discharged visualization, infrared thermography, and the single square voltage pulse method to demonstrate a close relationship between the increase in different forms of bioenergy and the increase in blood flow, two types of effects produced by Qigong and Tai Chi practice and also by heat and massage treatments.

What is the physiological significance of increased bioenergy resulting from Qigong Tai Chi practice? Recent research on the relationship of electrical field and wound healing has provided information that might be relevant to this important question. The skin of humans and animals is known to emit an electrical field of ~10 V/m under normal conditions, and the field goes up to ~100 V/m during wound healing (37-39). In a recent study, an externally applied D.C. electrical field of ~10-100 V/m was shown to enhance cell migration in the closing up of artificially created wounds in cell cultures (37). To investigate the molecular basis of this phenomenon, gene knockout experiments were conducted and it was found that the electrical effect on cell migration during wound healing involves the phosphorylation enzyme phosphatidylinositol-3-

Appendix

OH kinase, and the dephophorylation enzyme PTEN (abbreviation for Phosphatase Tensin Homology protein) (37). These two enzymes are known to be involved in many other cellular signaling pathways, including the ones that regulate the movement of cells towards chemical attractants (chemotaxis) (40, 41), and normal vascular development and tumor angiogenesis (42). Of particular interest to our research group is the fact that PTEN, first recognized as the product of a tumor suppressor gene (43), was named on the basis of its enzymatic activity and its structural homology with the gene for the cytoskeletal protein Tensin previously discovered in our laboratory (44). Thus, based on existing knowledge, we can propose a molecular and cellular model for how Tai Chi and Qigong practices can conceivably enhance healing in the body by stimulating cellular migration as a result of increased bioenergy especially in the form of electrical field. Clearly, the validity of this model needs to be tested in further experiments the future.

References

1) Lu, Z. (1997). Scientific Qigong Exploration. The Wonder and Mysteries of Qi. Amber Leaf Press, Malvern, PA.
2) Hintz, K.J., G.L. Yount, I. Kadar, G. Schwartz, R. Hammerschlag, and S. Lin. (2003). Bioenergy definitions and research guidelines. Alternative Therapies 9: A13-30.
3) Chen, K.W. (2004). An analytical review of studies on measuring effects of external Qi in China. Alternative Therapies 10: 38-50.
4) Luskin, F.M., K.A. Newell, M. Griffith, M. Holmes, S. Telles, E. DiNucci, F.F. Marvasti, M. Hill, K.R. Pelletier, and W.L. Haskell. (2000). A review of mind-body therapies in the treatment of musculoskeletal disorders with implications for the elderly. Altern. Therapies 6: 46-56.
5) Li, J.X., Y. Hong, and K. M. Chan. (2001). Tai Chi: physiological characteristics and beneficial effects on health (Review). Br. J. Sports Med. 35: 148-156.
6) Hong, Y., J.X. Li, and P.D. Robinson. (2000). Balance control, flexibility, and cardiorespiratory fitness among older Tai Chi practitioners. Br. J. Sports Med. 34: 29-34.
7) Thornton, E.W., K.S. Sykes, and W.K. Tang. (2004). Health benefits of Tai Chi exercise: improved balance and blood pressure in middle-aged women. Health Promotion International 19: 33-38.
8) Tsai, J.C., W.H. Wang, P. Chan, L.J. Lin, C.H. Wang, B. Tomlinson, M.H. Hsieh, H.Y. Yang, and J.C. Liu. (2003). The Beneficial effects of Tai Chi Chuan on blood pressure and lipid profile and anxiety status in a randomized controlled trial. J. Alt. Compl. Med. 9: 747-754.
9) Jones, B.M. (2001). Changes in cytokine production in healthy subjects practicing Guolin Qi Gong: A pilot study. BMC Complement Altern. Med. 1: 8.
10) Task Force of the European Society of Cardiology and the North American

Society of Pacing and Electrophysiology. (1996). Heart rate variability: Standards of measurement, physiological interpretation, and clinical use. Circulation 95: 1043-1059.

11) Lin, S., Z.Y. Shen, T. Ross, G. Chevalier, and K.M. Shu. (2006). Analysis of factors influencing the use of heart rate variability for evaluation of autonomic nervous function in mind/body and acupuncture research. J. Alt. & Compl. Med. 12: 223.

12) Lin, S., Z.Y. Shen, G. Chevalier, R. Srinivasan, T.P. Jung, and Z.P. Chen. (2004). Hi-tech measurements of physiological changes accompanying Chinese mind/body practices. In: Proceedings of the 10th Society of Chinese Bioscientists in America International Symposium, p.116.

13) Lin, S. Changes in mind-body functions associated with Qigong practice. (2004) J. Alt. & Compl. Med. 10: 200.

14) Jung, T.P., S. Makeig, M.J. McNeown, A.J. Bell, T.-W. Lee, and T.J. Sejnowski. (2001). Imaging brain dynamics using independent component analysis. Proceedings of the IEEE 89: 1107-1122.

15) Bonner, R.F., and R. Nossal. (1990). Laser Doppler Flowmetry. A.P. Sheppard and P.A. Oberg, Eds., Kluwer: Dordrecht, the Netherlands.

16) Lin, S., G. Chevalier, T. Ross, M. Nguyen, H. Lin, P. Lin, and Y. Lin. (2004). Comparison of bioenergy and physiological markers in Qigong and acupuncture research. J. Alt. & Compl. Med. 10: 1135.

17) Motoyama, H., Smith, W.T., and Harada, T. (1984). Pre-polarization resistance of the skin as determined by the single square voltage pulse method. Psychophysiology 21: 541-550.

18) Motoyama, H., D., M. Litt, B.S. Rake, and G. Chevalier. (1998). Bioenergy differences among races. Subtle Energies & Energy Medicine. 9: 101-131.

19) Lin, S., G. Chevalier, T. Ross, M. Nguyen, and H. Lin. (2006). Variability and specificity of the Single Square Voltage Pulse Method for measuring conductance at acupuncture points for mind-body research. J. Alt. & Compl. Med. 12: 210.

20) Cohen, S., and F.A. Popp. (1997). Biophoton emission of the human body. J. of Photochemistry & Photobiology B: Biology 40: 187-189.

21) Lin, S., G. Chevalier, H. Lin, T. Ross, and P. Lin. (2006). Measurement of biophoton emission with a single photon counting system. J. Alt. & Compl. Med. 12: 210-211.

22) Lin, S. and Z. Chen. (2007). A molecular and cellular model for benefits of increased bioenergy from Qigong/Tai Chi practice. J. Alt. & Compl. Med. 13: 905a.

23) K. Korotkov. (2002). Human Energy Field: Studies with Gas Discharge Visualization Bioelectrography. Backbone Publishing Co., Fair Lawn, New Jersey.

24)   http://www.ifpa-fitness.com/Fitness-Resources/Charts/Estimating_1rm_and_training_loads.htm

25) Lin, S., T. Ross, J. Guo, M. Kinoshita, M. Debbaneh, P. Wu, M. Meija, C. Le, E. Song, A. Lien, J. Hum, K. Perfecto, A. Sarkisyan, and M. Chen. (2007). Correlation of increased cutaneous blood flow with elevated bioenergy markers from Qigong/Tai Chi practice and heat/massage therapies. J. Alt. & Compl. Med. 13: 905b.

26) Li, F., P. Harmer, K.J. Fisher, E.McAuley, N. Chaumeton, E. Eckstrom, and N.L. Wilson. (2005). Tai Chi and fall reductions in older adults: A randomized controlled trial. J. Gerontology Series A: Biol. Sci. & Med. Sci. 60: 187-194.

27) Yeh, S.H., H. Chuang, L.W. Lin, C.Y. Hsiao, P.W. Wang, and K.D. Yang. (2007). Tai Chi Chuan exercise decreases A1C levels along with increase of regulatory T-cells and decrease of cytotoxic T-cell population in type 2 diabetic patients. Diabetic Care 30: 716-718.

28) Pedersen, B.K., A. Steenberg, and P. Schjerling. (2001). Exercise and interleukin-6. Curr. Opin. Hematol. 8: 137-142.

29) Pedersen, B.K., A. Steenbsberg, P. Keller, C. Keller, C. Fischer, N. Hiscock, G. van Hall, P. Plomgaard, and M.S. Febbraio. (2003). Muscle-derived interleukin-6: lipolytic, anti-inflammatory and immune regulatory effects. Pflugers. ArChiv.: Eu. J. Physiol. 446:9-16.

30) Jacobs, B.L., and C.A. Fornal. (1999). Activity of serotonergic neurons in behaving animals. Neuropsychopharmacology 21: 9S-15S.

31) Waldorp, T., F. Eldridge, G. Iwamoto, and J. Mitchell. (1996). Central neural control of respiration and circulation during exercise. In: Handbook of Physiology, Section 12, Exercise Regulation and Integration of Multiple Systems. L. Rowell, Ed., Oxford University Press, New York.

32) Bernardi, L., F. Keller, M. Sanders, P.S. Reddy, B. Griffith, F. Meno, and M.R. Pinsky. (1989). Respiratory sinus arrhythmia in the denervated human heart. J. Appl. Physiol. 67: 1447-55.

33) Felten, D.L. (2000). Neural influence on immune responses: underlying suppositions and basic principles of neural-immune signaling. Progress in Brain Research 122: 381-389.

34) Irwin, M.R., J.L. Pike, J.C. Cole, and M.N. Oxman. (2003). Effects of a behavioral intervention, Tai Chi Chih, on Varicella-Foster virus specific immunity and health functioning in older adults. Psychosomatic Medicine 65: 824-830.

35) Aftanas, L.I. and S.A. Golocheikine. (2001). Human anterior and frontal midline theta and lower alpha reflect emotionally positive state and internalised attention: high-resolution EEG investigation of meditation. Neuroscience Letters 310: 57-60.

36) Lee, M.S., B.H. Bae, H. Ryu, J.H. Sohn, S.Y. Kim, and H.T. Chung. (1997). Changes in alpha wave and state anxiety during ChunDoSunBup Qi-training in trainees with open eyes. Amer. J. of Chinese Med. 25: 289-299.

37) Zhao, M., B. Song, J. Pu, T. Wada, B. Reid, G. Tai, F. Wang, A. Guo, P. Walczysko, Y. Gu, T. Sasaki, A. Suzuki, J.V. Forrester, H. R. Blourne, P.N. Devreotes, C.D. McCaig, and J.M. Penninger. (2006). Electrical signals control wound healing through phophatidylinositol-3-OH kinase gamma and PTEN. Nature 442: 457-460.

38) Foulds, I. S. and A. T. Barker. (1983). Human skin battery potentials and their possible role in wound healing. Br. J. Dermatol. 109: 515–522.

39) McCaig, C. D., Rajnicek, A. M., Song, B. & Zhao, M. (2005). Controlling cell behaviour electrically: current views and future potential. Physiol. Rev. 85: 943–978.

40) Rickert, P., O.D. Weiner, F. Wang, H.R. Bourne, and G. Servant. (2000).

Leukocytes navigate by compass: roles of PI3K and its lipid products. Trends Cell Biol. 10: 466–473.

41) Iijima, M. and P. Devreotes. (2002). Tumor suppressor PTEN mediates sensing of chemoattractant gradients. Cell 109: 599–610.

42) Sasaki, H.K, P.A. Koni, M. Natsui, H. Kishimoto, J. Sasaki, N. Yajima, Y. Horie, G. Hasaqawa, M. Naito, J. Miyazaki, T. Suda, H. Itoh, K. Nakao, T.W. Mak, T. Nakano, and A. Suzuki. (2005). The PTEN/P13K pathway governs normal vasuclar development and tumor angiogenesis. Genes Dev. 19: 2054-2065.

43) Li, J., C. Yen, D. Liaw, K. Podsypanina, S. Bose, S.I. Wang, J. Puc, C. Miliaresis, L. Rodgers, R. McCombie, S.H. Bigner, B.C. Giovanella, M. Ittmann, B. Tycho, H. Hibshoosh, M.H. Wigner, and R. Parsons. (1997). PTEN, a putative protein tyrosine phosphatase gene mutated in human brain, breast, and prostate cancer. Science 275: 1943–1947.

44) Chuang, J.Z., D.C. Lin, and S. Lin. (1995). Molecular cloning, expression, and mapping of the high affinity actin-capping domain of Chicken cardiac tensin. J. Cell Biol. 128: 1095-1109.

Acknowledgements

We are grateful for the collaborations with members of the International Alliance for Mind-Body Signaling and Energy Research, particularly Drs. Zhong Yuan Shen, Ramesh Srinivazan, and Tzyy-Ping Jung. The research at the University of California, Irvine, was supported by the Joseph and Sou-Lin Lee Endowment for Traditional Chinese Medicine Research, the Lawrence S. Rockefeller Fund/Samueli Program for Energy Medicine Research, and institutional funds.

Simplified Personal History: B.S. and M.S. in Chemistry, and Ph.D. in Biological Chemistry from University of California, Los Angeles (1971). Professor (1974-1997) and Chairman (1983-1996) of Biophysics at Johns Hopkins University. Dean of Biological Sciences and Associate Vice Chancellor of Biological Initiatives at University of California, Irvine (1997-2002). Presently Professor of Cell Biology, Biomedical Engineering, and Integrative Medicine at University of California, Irvine. Practitioner and teacher of Kung Fu, Qigong, and Tai Chi for over 4 decades. Previously served as Co-Chair of the World Congress for Qigong (2004-2006) and Chair of the Think Tank on Biofield Energy Medicine of the National Center for Complementary and Alternative Medicine (2006). Present positions include membership on the Editorial Board of Journal of Alternative and Complementary Medicine, Editorial Board of Chinese Medicine, and the National Advisory Council for Complementary and Alternative Medicine for the National Institutes of Health.

Area of Research: Physiological and bioenergetic changes associated with Qigong and Tai Chi practices.

Published with author's permission.

Bibliography

Adler, Joseph A, "On Translating Taiji " Kenyon College June 2009; revised June 2012. Print

Bhikkhu, Buddhadasa. *Anapanasati* Trans. from the Thai Version by Bhikkhu Nagasena, Bangkok: Sublime Life Mission, 1976. Print

Blakeslee,Sandra, "What Other People Say May Change What You See" *New York Times* 28 June, 2005, Section F, Page 3. Print

Bi Yong Sheng, Sun Hua,Guo Yi Cao Zhenhua, Zhang MingQin, Zhang Bohua. *Chinese Qigong* Trans. Hu Zhaoyun, Shanghai PROC; Publishing House of Shanghai University of Traditional Chinese Medicine 1990. Print

Chang Po Tuan, *The Inner Teachings of Taoism* Trans. Thomas Cleary, Berkley: Shambhala, 2001. Print

Cheng Chien Bhikshu. *Sun-Face Buddha:The Teachings of Ma-Tsu and the Hung-Chou School of Ch'an* Fremont, CA: Jain Publishing Company, 2001. Print

Davis, Roy Eugene. *This is Reality* Lakemont, Ga: CSA Press, 1970. Print

Gia-Fu Feng and Jane English. *Tao Te Ching* Trans. Gia-Fu Feng and Jane English Vancouver: Vintage Books, 1977. Print

Hua-Ching Ni. *The Complete Works of Lao Tzu.* Santa Monica: Sevenstar Communications; Revised edition , 1995. Print

Jwing-Ming,Yang. *Qigong Meditation Embryonic Breathing* Boston: YMAA Publication Center 2003. Print

Kaptchuk,Ted J . *The Web That Has No Weaver* New York: Congdon &

Weed, 1983. Print

Lao Tzu. *Tao Te Ching*. Trans. Jonathan Star New York: Jeremy P. Tarcher / Putnam, 2001. Print

Liu I-Ming, *Awakening to the Tao* Trans. Thomas Cleary,Berkley: Shambhala, 1988. Print

Mah, Adeline Yen .*Watching the Tree*. New York: BroadWay Books, 2001. Print

Maharshi, Ramana. *The Spiritual Teaching of Ramana Maharshi* Berkeley: Shambhala, 1972. Print

Palmer, David A. *Qigong Fever* New York Columbia University Press, 2007. Print

Rosenberg, Marshall. *Compassionate Communication* Northwest Compassionate Communication web nwcompass.org/compassionate_ communication.html. 2012

Ruiz, Don Miguel. *The Four Agreements* San Rafael: Amber-Allen Publishing 1997. Print

Satir, Virginia. *The New Peoplemaking*. Los Altos. Science and Behavior Books Inc. 1988. Print

Sun Guangren, Liu Zhaochun,Li Hongbo,Yang SuQin,Chong GuiQin. *Health Preservation and Rehabilitation* Trans. Li Xuezhen, Sun Xigang, Sun Guangren, Zhang Peihua,Li Gouzhu, Li Caiping. Shanghai PROC; Publishing House of Shanghai University of Traditional Chinese Medicine, 1990. Print

Suzuki, D.T. *Mysticism: Christian and Buddhist* New York: George Allen & Unwin, 1957. Print

Tannen, Deborah. *I Only Say This Because I Love You,* New York Random House, 2001. Print

Wilber, Ken. *The Spectrum of Consciousness,* Wheaton, IL: Quest Books, 1989. Print

Wilhelm, Richard. *The Secret of the Golden Flower: A Chinese Book of Life* Trans. Cary F. Baynes, San Diego:Harcourt Brace Jovanovich Publishers edition, 1962. Print

Williamson, Marianne. *A Return To Love: Reflections on the Principles of A Course in Miracles.* New York: Harper Collins, 1992. Print

Wong, Eva. *Cultivating Stillness: A Taoist Manuel for Transforming Body and Mind.* Boston & London Shambhala, 1992. Print

Yu-Lan, Feng. *A History of Chinese Philosophy Vol.1 The Period of the Philosophers.* Trans. Derk Bodde. Princeton: Princeton University Press, 1952. Print

— Yu-Lan, Feng. *A History of Chinese Philosophy Vol.2 The Period of Classical Learning.* Trans. Derk Bodde. Princeton: Princeton University Press, 1953. Print

Yue, Tan. *The Principles of Tai Chi Chuan.* Shanghai Translation & Publishing Centre, Inc China, 1991. Print

Index

Richard Leirer

U

Unlocking the Frozen Gate 151

V

Virginia Satir 132

W

Wang, Zhang-Nan 143
Wave Hands Like Clouds 178
Waving Head and Tail 154
Weeping Willow Quivers in the Cool Breeze
        163
White Crane Flashes Its Wings 171
Wilbur, Ken 13
Wilhelm, Richard 42, 71
Wu Chi/Wuji 2
Wudang 144

X

Xia Dan Tien 90
Xiao Zhou Tian 94

Y

Yinjing 160
Yin and Yang 33
You Just Don't Understand 128
Yue 102
Yue Huanzhi 94
Yue Tan 91

Z

Zhang, San-Feng 142
Zhongqi 91
Ziran 101

232

24030150R00154

Made in the USA
San Bernardino, CA
08 September 2015